FEELING *the* WAY

FEELING
the WAY

TOUCH, QI GONG HEALING, AND
THE DAOIST TRADITION

ROB LONG

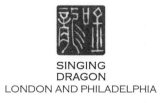

SINGING
DRAGON
LONDON AND PHILADELPHIA

First published in 2017
by Singing Dragon
an imprint of Jessica Kingsley Publishers
73 Collier Street
London N1 9BE, UK
and
400 Market Street, Suite 400
Philadelphia, PA 19106, USA

www.singingdragon.com

Library of Congress Cataloging in Publication Data
Names: Long, Rob, 1962- author.
Title: Feeling the way : touch, qigong healing, and the Daoist tradition /
 Rob Long.
Description: London ; Philadelphia : Singing Dragon, 2017. | Includes
 bibliographical references and index.
Identifiers: LCCN 2016016276 | ISBN 9781848192980 (alk. paper)
Subjects: | MESH: Therapeutic Touch--methods | Qi | Qigong--methods |
 Religion and Medicine
Classification: LCC RA781.8 | NLM WB 890 | DDC 613.7/1489--
dc23 LC record available at https://lccn.loc.gov/201601627

British Library Cataloguing in Publication Data
A CIP catalogue record for this book is available from the British Library

ISBN 978 1 84819 298 0
eISBN 978 0 85701 248 7

Printed and bound in Great Britain

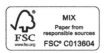

This book is dedicated to my daughter, Sally.
Whatever the Way may be, make it yours.

Contents

Acknowledgements

I would like to express my heartfelt thanks to everyone who has played a part in the creation of this book. In particular I'd like to acknowledge the contribution of Cassie Corby for her photography and patient encouragement throughout. Ann Burger, who graciously agreed to pose for some of the photographs, has also been a boundless source of support and enthusiasm, as has my dear friend and colleague, Shelagh Brady. Thanks are due too to Eilidh Moir for helping me initiate the project, and to Elaine Parsons for her meticulousness in proofreading the manuscript. Finally, I extend my endless gratitude to every single one of my patients over the last 20 years. Your kindness, fortitude and trust in indulging my exploration of the healing arts have been incalculable!

Disclaimer

The author and publisher of this material are not responsible in any way whatsoever for any distress or injury that may occur through reading or practising the exercises in this book.

Any healing art is safe only to the degree that it is practised safely. The author has gone to great lengths in this book to provide the reader with appropriate guidelines to ensure the wellbeing and safety of those in their care. If in individual cases there should be the slightest doubt as to whether or not to proceed, the author's recommendation at all times is to approach the patient's doctor first.

Note that none of the techniques outlined in this book are in any way a substitute for conventional health practices, medicines or any form of psychotherapy.

Preface

I live and work in the UK, part of a Western technological world remote in both time and culture from the sensibilities of ancient China. So distant are we, in fact, that it is sometimes hard to believe there could ever be any common ground between those two worlds. And yet, in the last 30 years or so, the influence of old China, and most particularly the teachings of those remarkable scholars, philosophers and proto-scientists – the Daoists – is making itself increasingly felt even here. Acupuncture, Qi Gong, Tai Chi, Chinese herbal medicine, Feng Shui and a whole host of other Daoist inspirations have become, if not exactly part of the warp and woof of everyday life for the majority of today's Westerners, then at least not utterly alien and therefore negligible phenomena. As the world becomes more and more magnetized by the irresistible pull of technology and commerce, so, too, does the ancient wisdom of the Dao begin increasingly to speak to us again, quietly, yet insistently. This should not surprise us – there can be no Yang without an answering Yin.

Why should this be so? Why is the gentle directness of the Daoist worldview so compelling to so many of us? The answer is simple. Any values with the power to strike a chord regardless of epoch, geography or culture do so because fundamentally they are *human* values, at which point all differences between us begin to fall away.

It was in the spirit of trying to capture the shared human values of Daoism and the modern world that I began to put together this book. Its subject is a new, distinctly unusual hands-on healing system that I have called Qi Sensitivity Healing, or QSH for short. It is very different from the more familiar style of healing practised in China today – External Qi Healing (EQH), a side-branch of Qi Gong.

QSH is 'mine' only in so far as I have taken the time to develop an entire range of healing techniques that I use in the clinic simultaneously with Acupuncture, Tui Na (Traditional Chinese Massage) and Qi Gong. It is designed to meld effortlessly with just about any complementary medicine modality, providing simple yet powerful tools for enhancing whatever therapy it is that one currently practises. There is no contradiction. And if you are not a therapist? The diligent practice of QSH will substantially increase your understanding of Qi, and therefore of all Daoist arts, in a very real, embodied way.

Whilst the specific techniques of QSH may be largely of my own invention, the rigorous medical discipline that underpins them is not. This belongs entirely to the Daoists and to the great body of theoretical knowledge that gave the world Traditional Chinese Medicine (TCM). What follows throughout the rest of this book is therefore, on the one hand, a detailed instruction manual and, on the other, a practical, kinetically based exploration of Daoist philosophy and science, in which your own body will be your laboratory. Potentially, we are all healers. I hope very much that this book will help you to embody that fundamental truth.

INTRODUCTION

It has been a challenging few weeks for this particular patient. Very little of what happens in her life seems within her control, or at least that's how she always depicts herself at our sessions. Today she is tired, anxious and on the threshold of becoming overwhelmed by her issues. She is, to use her own words, desperate for me to help her to 'just keep going'.

The Acupuncture I provide has served her well so far, always managing to get her 'back on track', at least so that she can function without the panic attacks and that general pervasive sense of dread she so often experiences. However, we both know from experience that Acupuncture is not the only thing that brings her back into balance…

So, whilst she relaxes on the treatment couch with the needles in situ, I ask if it will be alright for me to come and sit behind her, at the head of the couch, and perform my own brand of Daoist-inspired healing, Qi Sensitivity Healing (QSH). She's very familiar with this routine by now, so readily agrees. This, she says, is her favourite part of the entire treatment. I make myself comfortable and place my hands about six inches either side of her head, close my eyes and simply focus on my own posture and breathing. After a minute or two, everything starts to slow down, to become still, and so I switch my attention to the complex stream of sensations that I am now beginning to perceive with my hands. Meanwhile the patient continues to talk excitedly about the tribulations of the last few weeks, and whilst I am most definitely listening and even responding to her conversation, part of me is elsewhere entirely, deeply focused on the subtle manual sensations that are becoming clearer and more tangible by the second.

The Acupuncture she is receiving today is as formal as ever, a product of pulse taking, tongue examination and a diagnosis based on long experience and the painstakingly specific criteria of Traditional Chinese Medicine (TCM). This additional healing, although performed at exactly the same time as the Acupuncture, could not be more different. I am simply waiting for her energy field to tell me what to do, any intellectual appraisal of the situation deliberately 'switched off'. The answer is delivered soon enough in what I can only call a dawning of intuition, and before I've even had time to think about it, one of my hands has moved closer to her head and is hovering above an acupoint on her right temple known as Taiyang.[1] The corresponding point on her left side seems healthy enough, but there is definitely something indefinably 'not balanced' about right-sided Taiyang at this moment, and my hand has perceived this.

Without my asking it to, my hand now begins to make an involuntary circling motion that seems to amplify the sensations I'm receiving, but a few moments later it spontaneously adopts a different technique and begins to engage motionlessly with the acupoint from a few inches away. It now feels as if something cord-like is connecting my hand to the side of her head. I simply let the hand do whatever it wants to, for by now I know better than to try to analyse or direct this process. Although I have perceived this particular imbalance, I'm not actively going to do anything about it, other than watch and wait. Paradoxically, it is this very 'watching and waiting' that will produce the result we want.

By now the patient can feel something happening too. She giggles and tells me she always looks forward to this particular sensation and what, for want of a better phrase, she likes to call the 'lovely strangeness' of the healing experience. Then, in an instant, the energetic 'cord' that my hand has perceived quite suddenly comes away from the side of her head and disperses, almost exactly like a puff of smoke. At the same time, the acupoint I have been focused on starts to feel more alive, yet *neutral* again, and at this very moment the patient lets out a deep, contented sigh and seems to sink deeper into the fabric of the treatment couch. Of course, before I remove the needles I will re-examine her pulse, Chinese-style, and make sure that everything has harmonized in the way that was hoped for. Yet even before I do this I already know that today's will prove to have been a successful session – that deep sigh and spontaneous release of tension have said it all. The Acupuncture treatment has been enhanced, yet not in any way compromised. At the same time, merely by observing with great focus, the observer has somehow changed the outcome of this particular experiment. 'The Dao does nothing, and yet nothing is left undone.'

❖

Daoism, that beautiful, profound and often wilfully contradictory flower of ancient Chinese culture, is nothing if not durable. Walk into any high-street bookstore and you will be sure to find at the very least a handful of works that reference this specifically Chinese phenomenon. These range from weighty tomes on Oriental philosophy to 'how to' books on an entire range of Daoist-inspired (or, at the very least, Daoist-flavoured) subjects: Tai Chi, Qi Gong, Feng Shui, cookery, the arts (both martial and otherwise), business, diet and so on…

Perhaps this renewed interest in the Dao should not surprise us. After all, if there is one thing the ancient Daoists insisted on, it was the notion that everything in our universe ultimately moves in cycles, inexorably spiralling back to its primal origin in simplicity. Daoists called this 'returning to the source'.

In creating QSH, 'returning to the source' was exactly what I had in mind, and now I have also made it the central premise of this book. To that end I have hacked back some of the intellectual and theoretical thickets that often characterize Chinese Medicine as it is practised today, hoping that what lies beneath is nothing less than the unadorned truth of an encounter with another person's life force, their Qi. The watchword here is 'simplicity' – simplicity in how you treat your clients, if you are already a therapist, and also in how you regard yourself and what it means just to be human, whoever you may be.

Feeling the Way is aimed primarily, although not exclusively, at energy-based therapists who already have knowledge of Oriental Medicine. That is, acupuncturists, Shiatsu and Tui Na specialists and perhaps even teachers of Tai Chi, Qi Gong and Nei Gong. Masseurs, osteopaths, cranio-sacral and other bodywork professionals as well as martial artists might equally benefit to the extent that they are prepared to immerse themselves in the traditional Chinese milieu. Even if you are already trained in one or more Oriental Medicine modalities, you will most likely find a number of medical concepts here that are either new to you or at least presented in a very new light. And whilst the individual techniques of QSH might be mine, the entire mindset that underpins them is purely Daoist. One such Daoist value is utility, so it should come as no surprise that whilst this book is written to be interesting and entertaining, above all it's written to be useful. Its aim is to provide a specific skills set that you can use either as a stand-alone system or, far better still, *at exactly the same time as you are treating in your usual way*. All that you will read here is designed to be integrated seamlessly into your existing practice.

Undoubtedly, there is also a great deal presented in these pages that you will immediately recognize, particularly if you have been involved to any extent in Qi Gong or, better still, Nei Gong. However, this is emphatically not a textbook on either of these subjects. Whoever you are, to get the most from this book it is important to have not only a working knowledge of Acupuncture points and especially their precise locations, but also a reasonable grasp of the topography of the entire human energetic system, as understood by the ancient Chinese. You need to know the meridians and their preferred direction of flow. If you are not a therapist but merely a follower of Dao, there are a great many accessible textbooks available to furnish you with the technical information you will need, and some of these are listed in the 'Further Reading' section at the end of the book.

In these pages, therefore, you'll find a practical exploration of Daoism as expressed through the medium of hands-on healing, and also what we might call the medium of simplicity itself.

QSH is about effecting change through feeling, through kinetic sensation, and not merely through scholastic knowledge or professional technique. But be warned! QSH is nonetheless very much a discipline, with its own often rigorous demands. Daoism has always taken great delight in paradox, and QSH is just another manifestation of that tendency. Just as one needs to know the rules in order to break the rules, one also needs a great deal of self-cultivation to be able to just go with the flow. 'Simple' does not always equate to 'easy'!

QSH is therefore my own considered interpretation of certain fundamental Daoist principles, born of two decades of trial, error and the odd 'eureka' moment. I hope very much that you will find it of sufficient value to make you want to adopt it and absorb it into your current practice. It is, after all, straightforward, practical and effective. At the same time, it is most definitely more than a little mysterious. Exactly like the Dao itself!

How Qi Sensitivity Healing came about

In order to really grasp how QSH might differ from the wealth of other therapies now available in the West, I feel a little brief, but relevant, personal history might help.

I have been a practising acupuncturist in the UK since 1996. I am also a practitioner of Tui Na (Traditional Chinese Massage) and teach Qi Gong privately too. Mostly, however, even though it's not written anywhere on my business card, these days I think of myself as primarily a hands-on QSH healer with Acupuncture and Massage a mere 'front' for these more esoteric activities. I apply the hands-on approach whenever I feel it appropriate, which turns out to be most of the time. Most often this healing is applied whilst the client is already on the couch with needles in situ, or during a massage, and because the client and I are probably also having a very rewarding chat at the time, many of them do not even notice that they are being 'healed'. Overall, QSH has proved to be extremely popular and, more importantly, exceptionally useful in the clinic.

Like so many others, I myself first came to Daoism – specifically Daoist Acupuncture – as a patient. Well over 20 years ago I was working as a freelance writer in the hard-headed, somewhat frenzied world of advertising, and had allowed myself to become very ill indeed.

Inevitably, I eventually found myself being interviewed by a senior hospital consultant who blandly assured me I required radical, irreversible surgery. There was, he said, 'absolutely no other way'. I was terrified.

Somewhat in a panic, I decided instead to try Acupuncture as a last resort before submitting to the scalpel.

A friend had already suggested her acupuncturist, and the rest, as they say, is history. To the great surprise of everyone at the time, most especially myself, it turned out to be Acupuncture that was to produce a permanent, definitive cure, and in an amazingly short space of time.

I was now a convert, and, like all converts, I threw myself into the new world that had suddenly opened up before me with great zeal. I was seized with enthusiasm for gathering information on this seemingly bizarre and alien therapy that had effected such a remarkable healing in me. I signed up for Acupuncture college, enrolled in classes in Tai Chi and Qi Gong, qualified in Tui Na, and read voraciously on every aspect of Chinese culture, and most particularly Daoism. Something in that particular tradition resonated powerfully with me.

When I eventually found myself an established practitioner, my thirst for knowledge of all things Daoist or Chinese Medicine-related only seemed to increase. After all, I was now in a position where I was required to produce tangible results on a daily basis. My training was sound, but I wanted to do even better.

Everybody is a healer

Once again, I started to study. I went on as many courses as I could, and avidly read up on just about anything and everything that promised to flesh out my knowledge or provide me with an extra tool, some extra clinical skill. My reading was wide – everything from Chan Buddhism to meditation techniques and the internal martial arts. Nor did I restrict myself to purely Chinese material, but I immersed myself in the wisdom traditions and medical ideas of Japan, India, Tibet, and so on. I also talked to osteopaths, chiropractors, doctors, hands-on healers, dieticians – in fact anyone who might provide a valuable insight. I learned a great deal, but so far not even this wider exploration had fundamentally altered the way I approached my work in the clinic. That is, until I came across a Japanese healing modality that was very much en vogue at the time – Jin Shin Jyutsu.

Jin Shin Jyutsu has an allegedly ancient heritage and is clearly related to Chinese Medicine. It involves holding various parts of either a patient's body – or even one's own – the idea being that merely touching these points whilst focusing one's attention can produce a profound healing effect.

Now it is not my intention here to discuss the merits or otherwise of Jin Shin Jyutsu. I never formally trained in it, and it bears little resemblance to what eventually became QSH. However, inevitably I did experiment with the Japanese art on my own, and something very remarkable happened: *I discovered that I had healing hands.* For me this was one of those 'road to Damascus' moments, after which nothing could be quite the same.

From this perfectly thrilling realization it was but a short step to working out the obvious corollary: *everyone has healing hands*. And yes, that does mean you! Healing is not the exclusive province of 'special' individuals possessed of some mystical power. It is a basic human ability and the birthright of us all, even if it does lie largely dormant in the general populace. Whatever is dormant can be awoken. The Dao isn't merely something one talks about or reads about – the Dao is in your own hands, quite literally! I didn't take any of this on board as an article of faith, of course, but put it to the test in every way I could. The result, after many years of trial and error, was the creation of the simple, direct and Daoist-inspired healing system I now call Qi Sensitivity Healing.

QSH is based solidly on the traditional Daoist virtues of:

- simplicity

- intuition

- spontaneity

- awareness.

In clinical terms, QSH lends itself to healing[2] on all levels at which the human condition presents itself, that is:

- physically

- emotionally/psychologically

- spiritually.[3]

If you are seeking to augment your existing therapy, to develop a greater feel for Qi, or simply to embody in your daily life some of the breathtaking philosophical insights of the ancient Chinese, this book has been written to help you do just that. It combines an exploration of key Daoist ideas and technologies with step-by-step instructional exercises graded from child's play to the distinctly challenging. It contains everything you need to practise QSH. To heal others is a privilege; to do it well is nothing less than a joy.

Notes

1. Locations for all the acupoints mentioned in this book are given in the appendix.

2. I define the word 'healing' as 'that which brings about welcome change in a human being'. It does not necessarily imply 'curing', as some conditions are clearly not amenable to cure, such as terminal illness. However, quality of life is always the main consideration, whether that means a reduction in physical pain, or helping someone to find the peace to die with courage and dignity. It is all 'healing'.

3. 'Spiritual' strikes me as a much-abused word! In the context of QSH it refers to the deeper, potentially more transformative aspects of a human being, those qualities that can give a person connection with others and with life itself. There is no implication here of anything transcendental, although, admittedly, some very remarkable experiences do sometimes occur during QSH sessions.

Chapter 1

WHAT IS A DAOIST?

As discussed in the Introduction, Qi Sensitivity Healing (QSH) was created to be a practical example of 'Daoism in action'. Yet before we can fully embody that idea, it might be important to define exactly what we mean by the terms 'Daoism' and 'Daoist'. I am going to focus almost exclusively on whatever insights into the Daoist mind are immediately relevant to the practice of QSH. However, strict definitions, like the Daoists themselves, are sometimes elusive…

I do not feel myself particularly qualified to provide any in-depth, historical or philosophical treatise on Daoism; I leave that to academics. There are already many superb works on the subject, and besides, for our purposes here, a weighty scholastic appraisal is not really necessary. One thing that we do need to understand about Daoism, however, is that it is not one single, unified entity and never was. The history of China is long and tortuously complex.

Indeed, the Chinese can rightly lay claim to having the oldest unbroken civilization in the world. Despite, for example, numerous civil wars, invasion by the Mongols, Westerners and the Japanese, endless regime changes and the seismic upheavals of the Communist era, China has always managed to remain quintessentially itself. Unfortunately, when it comes to attempting even a thumbnail sketch of a phenomenon like Daoism, the very size and antiquity of

China become something of an impediment in themselves. By this I'm suggesting that over the millennia Daoism has meant a great many different things to a great many people. It has been, by turns, a magical, shamanic practice, a form of alchemy, an early science, a spiritual philosophy based on close observation of Nature, a state religion,[1] a catalyst of political rebellion,[2] and even a means of exerting military control via its own Daoist army![3]

The practical and mystical become one

So, if it is a given that Daoists are hard to pin down to any particular orthodoxy or predictable type of behaviour, it still benefits us to take a brief look at those salient features of Daoism that might still prove relevant to us as QSH healers.

Of the multiplicity of people who have understood themselves in so many different ways to be 'Daoist', we are really concerned here with but one major grouping. These are, of course, the so-called Philosophical Daoists of classical Chinese antiquity, long before Daoism became a religion or political tool. It was they who created the mindset personified by such sages as Chuang Tzu and Lieh Tzu and most notably by Lao Tzu, venerable author of the *Classic of the Way*, the *Dao De Jing*. It is the Philosophical Daoists who have provided the conceptual framework, both for QSH and for this book. These are those very same rugged individualists who gave us Acupuncture, Tai Chi, Qi Gong and Chinese herbalism, to name but a few of their inspirations. They are the ones who initiated what was arguably the world's first ever 'scientific' revolution by testing their many hypotheses and drawing their conclusions from meticulous trial and error. Lacking modern technology, their yardsticks were their own bodies and minds, and systematic observation of the natural world was de rigeur. These ancient Daoist men and women explored in painstaking detail every imaginable avenue of life, from warfare to medicine, from the wilder shores of sexuality to transcendent spirituality. They were both rebels and bastions of society, hermits and landed aristocracy, fearsome soldiers and embodiments of peace and compassion. They were simultaneously playful and contrary, and yet deadly serious in their self-discipline and determination to discover all that life had to offer. They epitomized passionate, aware living that was sometimes so far beyond the pale of Chinese orthodoxy that people often thought them literally mad.

Understanding the world through personal experience

Philosophical Daoism engaged the mind in a rigorous, objective way that we could call 'proto-scientific'. Close, detailed observation of Nature and the mechanisms that underpinned it was of the greatest importance. However, at the same time this secular movement was nothing if not *mystical*. Here I define the word 'mystical' as something that encourages a direct, personal experience of the ineffable. This is, of course, quite the opposite of what we could term 'religion', which strongly implies beliefs that are received, and not necessarily based on any kind of personal experience at all. The Philosophical Daoists were having none of this. So even though they conceived of the Dao as the deeply mysterious, undifferentiated spiritual force that underlay the fabric of reality, nothing was to be taken at face value. Everything must be tested, experienced at first hand. We might call this a kind of 'scientific spirituality', perhaps an oxymoron to the average Westerner, but not to a Daoist.

This insistence of first-hand experience is also one of the foundations of QSH. QSH deals exclusively with Qi, the subtle realms. Accordingly, it is all too easy to convince ourselves that we are feeling something significant when we are not. Our egos often require particular outcomes, and without clear focus our kinetic sensitivities become confused. To avoid this, one needs only to remember the following maxim: 'Believing Is Seeing'. Don't believe anything – feel it for yourself. You will never become an effective healer if you cannot learn empirically. And please don't worry; amongst other things, this book is a training manual for how to perceive Qi clearly and decisively. In Chinese, the term Ting Jing translates as something like 'listening to Qi', and this ability to listen is the primary skill of a QSH healer. Whenever we are working with Qi, we are engaging simultaneously with mystery and with earth-bound practicality. This is a very Daoist approach to life, and demands a level of disciplined sensitivity in which lack of clarity and wish fulfilment have no place.

The very real, kinetic sensations that need to be perceived and balanced when applying QSH are almost certainly best understood by first studying ourselves. The exercises that follow in this chapter will help you to start to settle into this way of thinking. This is entirely in line with traditional Daoist methods of teaching energy arts. In *Heavenly Streams*, Nei Gong master Damo Mitchell comments: 'The ancient approach to Chinese Medicine differs greatly from the modern way of learning. Students are encouraged to first explore the nature of their own energy system prior to beginning their work on other people's' (Mitchell 2013, p.21).

How else, then, might philosophical Daoism be relevant to QSH? Non-forcing, clearly perceiving the flow of events, individualism, spontaneity, minimal intervention, compassion – these are all traditional values that inform the Daoist worldview and manifest in multiple ways in Daoist arts, from sculpture and politics right through to hands-on healing. Such values manifest, for instance, in familiar Daoist concepts such as Wu-Wei (acting appropriately with minimum force or effort), and what we could call 'the pursuit of naturalness'. QSH, like Daoism, is concerned with bypassing the rational, judicial mind, and returning instead to a finely tuned, intuitive state of being. Each of these elements is embedded in the practice of QSH, and will be discussed at some length elsewhere in this book.

In the meantime, perhaps we should set the ball rolling by starting to develop our relationship with our own Qi.

Exercise 1.1: Child's play

The following preliminary exercise is often, quite literally, a children's game in China. Anybody who has even the most passing acquaintance with Qi Gong will almost certainly have encountered it too. Due to its very simplicity it is often overlooked, or treated merely as a means of energizing the hands prior to more serious work. In QSH, however, it is to be regarded as a core skill. Please don't skip it! Far more demanding exercises will inevitably follow in this book, but, even so, unless you are already a distinguished Qi Gong master, I strongly recommend that you return often to this particular 'game'. It reveals its hidden depths slowly and over time, and will enhance your healing abilities in direct proportion to how often you practise it.

The usefulness of a skill does not always lie in its complexity. For example, whilst I was studying the internal–external martial art of Wing Chun, it was demonstrated to me how all the essentials of that entire system are actually secretly embedded in the preliminary 'warm-up'. Anybody too eager to move on to more advanced techniques would have utterly failed to notice this, and been the poorer for it. A similar principle applies here. And quite frankly, this exercise is a great deal of fun!

So, I'd like you just to sit or stand comfortably and allow yourself a few slow, deliberate breaths.

Please don't try to clear your mind at this stage – or at any other stage for that matter. Even highly experienced meditators find this difficult, and you might just be setting yourself up for failure, with all its attendant frustration and tension. Tension is the last thing we want here.

Instead, let's give the mind something to do.

Hold your hands apart with the palms facing each other, about one foot apart (see Figure 1.1). There is no need to be more precise than that at this stage. Now, focus your attention on your hands. If it helps, it's fine to close your eyes, although later on in clinical practice you'll definitely have more awareness if you keep them open.

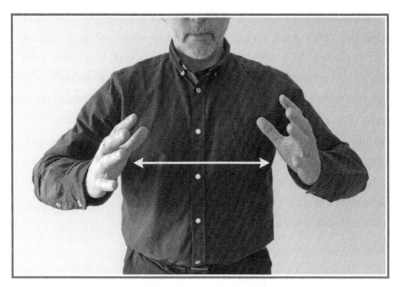

Figure 1.1: Beginning hand posture

Begin to move your hands slowly apart, to a distance of, say, shoulder-width. Just note exactly how that feels, throughout your entire body, but most specifically in your hands. Now, equally slowly and with as much unbroken attention as you can muster, bring the hands back together until your palms are almost touching, but don't let them actually make contact.

Remember: this is just a 'game' at this stage, so the more lightheartedly you treat the entire thing, the more you should gain from it. Relaxation is everything.

Keep pulling the hands apart and closing them again. Has the quality of sensation in your hands begun to change yet? What precisely are you feeling there? Maybe nothing in particular, maybe a great deal. Right now it doesn't matter; we're simply exploring, so keep going for a minute or two.

Finally, bring the hands together to within about four or five inches, palms still facing.

Again, do not let them touch if you can avoid it. Now start to 'roll' the hands, as if there were something about the size and shape of a tennis ball between them (see Figure 1.2).

Experiment with letting the hands rotate in different directions, whatever feels good. What is happening now? What sensations are you feeling? Play with this 'tennis ball' for a little while, and when you've had enough, simply let your hands fall away from each other and return to a gentle observation of your breathing. Whilst you're doing that, try to notice if anything else about you has changed. For example, are you more relaxed, clearer-headed, hotter, cooler, calmer, more energized? In a way it really doesn't matter what you are feeling, so long as you are feeling something that previously you were not. Right now, the vital thing is simply that to the best of your ability *you have noticed in great detail whatever is happening.*

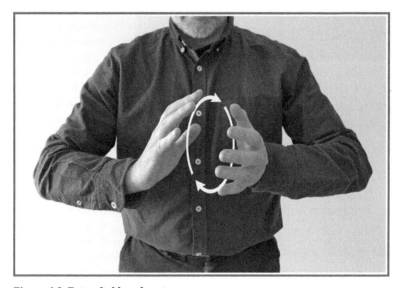

Figure 1.2: Extended hand posture

So was that fun? Some of you will have performed this particular exercise many times before – it is pretty basic – but if you haven't, it can be quite a revelation.

Limitations of language

By now you may have come to realize that at no point in this book am I going to tell you what you should or should not be feeling. We are all unique individuals, with unique wiring, and so there is no 'should' implicit in any of this. There is also the problem of language. Any words we can employ to try to describe different qualities of Qi will inevitably be inadequate for the task. To respectfully misquote Lao Tzu, 'The Qi that can be spoken of is not the true Qi.' Qi is literally indescribable, but for the purposes of this book, I have done my best to convey a range of subjective sensations.

Then there is the issue of our innate human uniqueness. I am not you, and so I have no idea of *precisely* what will occur for you. Having said that, from my experience of working with Qi Gong students there are certain sensations that most of us seem to share in common, and so I'm going to tentatively suggest that in doing the above exercise you might well have felt something akin to 'solidity' between your hands. I might also speculate that this slightly dense 'something' might have struck you as vaguely spherical and have 'magnetic' properties of attraction and repulsion. Perhaps there was warmth and tingling too, and this might even have registered itself in other parts of your body. Possibly you felt calmer, or more grounded after the exercise…

Again, it's vital to understand that there is absolutely no right or wrong to any of this. Some people will feel a great deal, others less so. Some people experience epiphanies; others really have to work at it. (Despite the discovery that I could heal others, I still don't regard myself as a 'natural' when it comes to perceiving Qi, so I am definitely one of those who have had to work hard to develop my sensitivities!) Thus far I have yet to meet anyone who feels nothing at all during these exercises, but if you do happen to be that person, please don't worry – the sensitivity will come, I promise. As I've noted in the Introduction to this book, after a great deal of observation it is my firm belief that simply everybody can learn to develop healing hands. This is a normal human ability, but in many of us it needs to be awakened and carefully cultivated thereafter. The exercises that follow in the coming chapters will teach you how to do this, and will become progressively more subtle, powerful and clinically useful. As we go more deeply into our exploration of Dao, they will also become progressively more challenging.

Notes

1. During the Han dynasty, approximately concurrent with the birth of Christianity, Daoism became an official Chinese religion, based on the worship of Lao Tzu as a god. One wonders what the venerable old philosopher would have made of that had he been alive to see it!

2. In AD 184, as many as 350,000 Chinese rose up in rebellion at what they saw as the suppression of Daoism. Meanwhile, throughout China's history, Daoists have been engaged in, for example, teaching martial arts skills to peasants to enable them to defend themselves against tyrannical landlords and rulers. At many times in China's past, Daoists have been viewed with suspicion by ruling elites who saw them as a potential threat to the status quo. Perhaps with good reason!

3. In the 2nd century AD, Chang Heng, son of the originator of the Daoist Heavenly Masters sect, was gifted an army by the despotic Duke of Chou. This is not how most modern Westerners conceive of Daoist behaviour.

Chapter 2

BREATHE!

In this chapter we're going to take a much closer look at how one crucial element can positively affect our capabilities as healers. This is the science of breathing. As we shall see, 'science' is most certainly the appropriate word here, and this particular study has an extremely long track record in the Far East.

For several millennia, people in China, Tibet, India and other Asian countries have carried out a thorough and profound investigation into the subject of using the breath. It was realized from early times that consciously altering or controlling how we breathe could have ramifications for almost every aspect of life. For instance, there are specific breath control techniques for everything from meditation to martial arts to making love. A multiplicity of specialized techniques exists for, to cite a few more examples, enhancing longevity, optimizing scholastic performance, achieving spiritual bliss and, of course, manifesting powerful healing abilities.

Whilst this Asian focus on uses of the breath undeniably produced a great variety of (occasionally contradictory) opinion, often generated by ethnic, religious or cultural differences, it nonetheless gave the world a vast compendium of knowledge, almost all of which is broadly in accord. For example, the Indian sage Patanjali, founder of the famous Pranayama school of yogic breathing, gives a lot of emphasis to holding, counting and releasing the breath in highly specialized ways. This produces remarkable results, although it does require a considerable level of focus and effort, at least at first. There was throughout history a great deal of intellectual interchange and what we could call 'cross-fertilization' between China and other nearby lands – India and Tibet in particular. So it is hardly surprising that some Daoist techniques are very similar to methods such as Pranayama, whose origins lie quite obviously in those other countries. Despite this, I would argue that the majority of Daoist ideas on breathing are homegrown. This is because they tend mostly to gravitate towards the other end of the breathing spectrum – in other words, where the breath is simply observed or gently guided with the least amount of force possible. This is not to imply any qualitative difference between Daoist and non-Daoist approaches to breathing; each system arose as a creative solution to a specific challenge, and each either passed the test of time or fell into disuse long ago.[1] The point is that whatever its origin, each style was effective for the purpose it was designed for, and each cultivated the ability to breathe consciously and with control. As QSH healers, we will need to be ever mindful of this.

Meanwhile, the Daoists themselves were busy creating or adapting dozens, if not hundreds, of breath cultivation methods, and it is well nigh impossible to isolate a single, definitive strand that we could call 'Daoist breathing'. What we can say with confidence, however, is that all these practices are simply variations on the same recurrent theme: the notion that the breath is a highly effective tool – perhaps *the* tool – for uniting our innate resources.

For our purposes as healers, the Daoist virtues of *simplicity and utility* are once again what we need to be emphasizing here. For us, this means consciously entering a state where ease, spontaneity and naturalness can arise, all by themselves. There must be no forcing. In addition, we must aim to develop only those methods that *our own experience* in the clinic tells us are useful. Keep it simple! This is certainly the foundation of the QSH approach.

Breathing as a technology

I teach various Daoist breathing techniques as a matter of course to my Qi Gong students, and have also attempted to pass on some of the simpler ones to many of my clients, whenever I felt they might benefit. I use the word 'attempted' advisedly, as far from everybody is open to these ideas at first. Therein lies the nub of the problem: most Westerners are utterly unaware that their breathing is unhealthy. What's more, here in the West there is absolutely no cultural orientation that leads people to believe that changing how they breathe could have a positive impact on their lives. After all, barring some kind of respiratory condition, everybody already knows how to breathe, don't they? We've done it all day long ever since we took that first breath as a baby.

If one looks at breathing as a purely unconscious act whose sole purpose is to bring an adequate supply of oxygen into the body, then yes, of course everyone already knows how to breathe. In the Orient, however, breathing is both a *technology* and a *spiritual discipline*. In *A Path with Heart*, Buddhist meditation master Jack Kornfield comments: 'Every place we feel the breath in our body can come alive with subtle vibrations, movement, tingles, flow. The steady power of our concentration shows each part of our life to be in change and flux, like a river' (2002, p.62). Here in the West, the majority of people are blind to such an alien notion, at least at first. (According to my observations, that also includes many therapists!) So, as Qi Gong master B.K. Frantzis is often heard to say in his seminars, 'If you're going to learn just one thing from Daoist energy arts, learn the breathing.'

What is it, then, about our breathing that as QSH healers we might wish to improve on, and why? Before we can fully answer this question, it is helpful first to examine some of the structural and biochemical dynamics of breathing. By recognizing what could be called a 'healthy norm', we can begin to see how we might be deviating from that norm. I'm going to look at this issue from the perspective of both Western and Chinese medicines.

Take a look, if you can, at a pet cat, dog or horse, or perhaps at a baby or pre-school child. Which part of their body is most engaged in the breathing process? Assuming your subject is healthy and not suffering from stress, it should be obvious that it is the lower abdomen that is moving the most during breathing. It expands like a balloon on inhalation and naturally collapses back in on itself during the out-breath. Meanwhile, the chest tends to remain fairly static, although, crucially, not rigid, as there is some lateral movement of the ribcage. This idea that the breath should principally expand and contract the lower abdomen can come as quite a surprise to many people. It's certainly not how they're breathing on a day-to-day basis, and when they attempt it, they can find it quite challenging. In fact, a great many of my patients are simply unable to do it! Perhaps this is a measure of how far modern society has taken us from our natural inclinations; after all, abdominal respiration was almost certainly what every one of us employed in our infancy. This natural method of breathing, with a relaxed and mobile lower abdomen compared with a relatively immobile thorax, has evolved as a simple result of the body's oxygen requirements.

The diaphragm, that large sheet of muscle that stretches between the lungs and the abdominal cavity, is required to rise and fall freely and smoothly in order to optimize oxygen intake. In so doing it also assists the heart and vascular system in moving blood around the body – hence its unofficial name, the 'second heart'. Diaphragmatic movement also gently massages the lower internal organs. Ideally, then, the diaphragm is pulled downwards effortlessly on inhalation. (This is an automatic movement, and should not require our conscious control if we are healthy breathers any more than we should need to tell our heart how and when to pump our blood.) The up-down motion of the diaphragm not only provides the optimal amount of surface area for gaseous exchange via the lungs' alveoli, but also creates a vacuum into which air will inevitably flow. Again, this should require no conscious effort on our part. On exhalation the diaphragm releases upwards, space within the chest cavity decreases accordingly, and carbon dioxide-laden air is naturally let out.

Achieving this unforced, easy motion is, of course, why the Daoists usually insist that we 'allow' a breath, rather than the more pro-active Western concept of 'taking' a breath. We don't need to be taking anything here; it's enough simply to get ourselves out of the way of genetically hard-wired mechanical processes and our body will 'breathe' quite happily all on its own. How at odds this is with the usual Western idea that a 'deep breath' is one in which we consciously try to fill the chest cavity to capacity! Try it now, and just observe how it makes you feel. Tight? Restricted? Anxious even? Does your heart speed up? Is your diaphragm even able to move at all? Now imagine being compelled to breathe in this manner all day long. Unfortunately, that is precisely what is happening for a significant proportion of the population. Medically, it's called hyperventilation syndrome, and quite simply it wreaks havoc.

Under normal circumstances, all breathing should ideally occur through the nose, the sophisticated internal structure of which is ideally designed both for warming air before it enters the lungs and for filtering out unwelcome particles.

So much for the physical mechanism. Western science has also studied the biochemical effects of breathing. This research has shed light not only on the pathogenesis of certain medical conditions, but also on the general *emotional* repercussions of poor breathing. The biochemistry is a little complex, but, essentially, chest breathing changes the chemical balance of our blood, making it more alkaline and less able to release its payload of oxygen. Two organs that require a particularly rich oxygen supply are the heart and the brain, and it's not hard to imagine what might ensue if these are deprived for any length of time. In terms of our emotional and psychological state, chest breathing can activate the sympathetic nervous system, the famous 'fight or flight' response. In other words, it primes us for a highly stressful situation, one in which, as far as the body is concerned, we are in mortal danger.

Again, imagine living with this level of stress every day, and what that could do to your sense of wellbeing. Needless to say, many, many people already do live like that.

It's not all gloom, though. Engaging the diaphragm in a relaxed way has been shown to have the exact opposite effect to chest breathing. Adrenalin and other stress hormones are de-emphasized, the heart beats less forcefully, blood pressure drops, the blood becomes less alkaline, and muscles relax as the parasympathetic nervous system takes over. In this way – purely through the manner in which we breathe – chaos or calm can be brought to the mind and body.

The ancient Chinese paradigm

The traditional breathing paradigm from China does not contradict the Western model, even if superficially it looks quite different. For instance, whilst the ancient Chinese did not have a precise formulation of the germ theory of disease, they most certainly understood that pathogens could enter the body via the nasal passages. These are the Xie Qi, 'pernicious or toxic influences', a term that also embraces the idea of purely *energetic* pathogens, inimical vibratory frequencies of Qi that could disrupt the body's internal coherence. The environmental frequencies collectively known as 'Cold' and 'Damp' were seen as the worst of these with regard to the health of the Lung, giving rise to the Chinese idea that the Lung was the 'tender organ', in need of greater care and protection.

When it comes to diaphragmatic breathing, called by the Chinese 'abdominal breathing', the Daoists did indeed broadly concur with modern Western findings, but typically also added their own unique observations. These are based solidly on the Oriental concept of the 'energetic anatomy', and as such have no

Western counterpart. As QHS practitioners, this is the aspect of breathing that should interest us the most.

Before examining this, let's take a break now to do something more experiential.

Exercise 2.1: Breathing with the belly

Sit or stand in a comfortable position. Allow yourself to breathe in whatever way is normal to you at the moment. DO NOT try to alter how you breathe. In fact, don't try to alter anything at all, as right now we are simply making an assessment, not an attempt to improve anything.

This exercise is about *noticing*. Noticing really is going to be a principal skill when you come to heal others.

Now, be aware first of all whether you are breathing through your mouth or your nose. Again, don't attempt to change things – just acknowledge what you find.

Can you feel the air penetrating? What does it feel like? How deep into the lungs does it go? What is its temperature?

Is it easy to allow the breath into your body, or is there some resistance or tension? If so, is this mainly physical, or is your mind playing a part too? Where exactly is the tension? In the throat, the ribs, the sternum? Is there any sense of obstruction or discomfort at the solar plexus?

What is your chest doing as you breathe? Do your ribs move? What about the space between your shoulder blades – is there any expansion or contraction there? Can you feel any movement, however slight, in your lower back?

The lower abdomen – is it moving? If so, does that feel easy or forced? Are you aware of what your diaphragm is doing? Can it move? And your belly – does it balloon out slightly when you breathe in, or are you drawing it in instead? Don't judge, just watch, just notice.

Now focus on increasingly less tangible aspects of your breathing. Can you feel anything that might be a sign of Qi, such as warmth, tingling or some more refined sense of 'movement' within the body? What exactly is that like, and where is it? Try to be very specific. Maybe you feel nothing yet. That's okay too.

What about your feet? Can you feel any sensation there that you were previously unaware of, and is there any sense of 'connection' with the ground? Do the hands feel alive or merely neutral?

Emotions? Thoughts? Insights? Spontaneous visual imagery? You might be experiencing all or none of this. It doesn't matter; for now we're still just noticing.

Finally, return to your lower abdomen. If you can, just let your mind gently rest there, doing nothing in particular and simply observing any subtle changes in your experience of that part of your body. As a healer, you will be spending a significant portion of your time just abiding in your lower abdomen, but for now don't worry if your mind wanders a little. We are eventually going to train our focus in this respect.

Continue this exercise for as long as you wish. I suggest at least five minutes. Compare your experience right in this moment with what your breathing was telling you at the very start of the exercise. Has anything changed? What? Again, don't judge, just observe and be honest with yourself.

When you're ready, gently bring the session to a close.

Compared with Qi Gong or other internal disciplines you may already know, this exercise is extremely uncomplicated – beginner's stuff. Don't be fooled, and please don't be impatient. In QHS this is once again a core skill that we are training here: *the ability simply to notice without judgement.* What we notice will become more useful and more profound every time we practise the exercise, and will have huge implications for us once we begin to lay hands on others.

Breathing and the Dan Tien

Anyone with a knowledge of Daoist arts will know about the Dan Tien, which translates into English as the 'elixir field'.

Strictly speaking, there are three Dan Tien, located respectively in the lower abdomen, the centre of the chest and the forehead. When we speak of the Dan Tien, we are really using a shorthand for the lower of the three, located deep within the core of the body, approximately two finger-widths below the navel, and on a line directly above the acupoint Hui Yin (CV 1), at the centre of the perineum. The precise location varies a little between individuals, as the Dan Tien can actually sometimes be found closer to the spine. There is only one way to find out where yours is, of course, and that is to begin to *notice* it whilst you are breathing! For many of us, that can take a little perseverance, but it's definitely a major step in your progress.

The term 'elixir field' refers to the internal cultivation of more and better-quality Qi. It's a rather agrarian metaphor that encourages us to look at the Dan Tien as a 'field' (actually a swirling ball of energy) in which the elixir of health and longevity can be 'grown'. This is, of course, a vital aim in all Daoist internal arts, and you will probably already be very familiar with the concept. Every time we consciously breathe into the Dan Tien, we are harmonizing, stabilizing and increasing our store of Qi. On this model it is a kind of battery. We could also look at all three Dan Tien as step-up/step-down transformers, passing energies up and down the body. The most dense energetic vibrations emanate from the lower Dan Tien, Jing (essence) and as they ascend are increasingly rarefied into Qi (life force) and Shen (intellectual and spiritual energy). This is the famous theory of the 'Three Treasures', and as such tends to be very well known, needing no further discussion here.

Yet another familiar function of Dan Tien is its ability to stimulate the spinal acupoint Ming Men (GV 4). Ming Men translates as 'gate of vitality' and has a conspicuous energizing and revitalizing effect on the energy body as a whole, with a particularly close relationship with Kidney energy. Again, it is the breath that catalyses this feature of the system.

However, there is another, equally crucial aspect to the Dan Tien that is sometimes overlooked. Complementing the battery-transformer metaphors described above, the lower Dan Tien must also be seen as the body's most important energy *pump*. In the average human being, the swirling ball of energy rotates every 24 hours, synchronized with the activity of the earth's magnetic core to which every living creature is 'plugged in'. This rotation within the lower abdomen is the principal means by which Qi is pumped throughout the meridian system. The importance of this cannot be overstated and has particular resonance for hands-on healers.

Having perceived all of these natural functions within their own bodies, the ancient Daoists characteristically wished to improve on Nature's basic model, as they did with just about everything they encountered. So how could we improve on this innate pumping function?

The answer is simple: by consciously breathing into the Dan Tien! Looked at this way, one's breathing suddenly becomes far more important than even Western science acknowledges.

Let's put that to the test, with another exercise.

Exercise 2.2: Letting the breath wake up the hands

Assume a comfortable position, sitting or standing.

Now bring your hands to within approximately three to four inches of each other, palms facing. Do not let the hands touch.

Try once more to get the feeling of a 'tennis ball' of Qi between your palms by gently rotating them as you did in Exercise 1.1.

At the same time, consciously but without any undue effort, breathe into your lower abdomen, being particularly aware of the approximate theoretical location of your Dan Tian.

Divide your attention equally between the hands and the belly – you can do it.

Notice what has happened to your hands when you breathe this way. Again, I'm not going to tell you what to feel, but I am going to suggest that you might have experienced a huge difference in the amount and quality of sensation in your hands once you started to breathe with gentle awareness into the abdomen. It's quite likely that your hands suddenly 'came alive' on an entirely new level. And if they didn't, fear not! It will come with time and practice. It is precisely this sense of aliveness that we are going to harness in our QSH healing work.

Exercise 2.3: A suggested breathing routine

It's very important in Daoism never to strain, struggle or force any desired outcome. Much better results will come from gentle, good-humoured perseverance. So please don't read the following as a set of rigid rules that you must adhere to doggedly. Just do your best and have fun with it, and if you're already an adept, it still doesn't hurt to remind yourself of some fundamentals!

Adopt a good sitting or standing posture – not too stiff, not too slack. (There is much more about posture in Chapter 3.)

Place the tip of your tongue gently against the roof of your mouth and keep it there.

Breathe calmly and slowly through the nose, noting all that you may experience as you do so.

Keep your sternum reasonably still, but see if your ribs might want to expand out to the sides when you inhale.

Ask the space between your shoulder blades to expand slightly sideways too.

Suggest to your lower back that it might want to expand by a tiny amount as well.

At the same time, notice your lower belly ballooning out effortlessly as you inhale. Force nothing.

Without holding the breath in any way, smoothly exhale, observing how the belly, ribs and lower back return naturally to their former positions.

Throughout this entire exercise, keep at least a portion of your mind peacefully anchored on the lower Dan Tien.

See if you can allow the entire breathing process to be slow, smooth and silent.

Notice anything and everything that you perceive whilst breathing by this method.

For the remainder of the exercises in this book, try to keep to this basic but immensely powerful approach to breathing, even if you already know more sophisticated methods. It will pay off.

Notes

1. Pranayama is at least 2250 years old, and was itself a development of a far earlier body of knowledge in India. Some would argue that Tibetan techniques are the oldest of all, although that might be hard to prove.

Chapter 3

THE BASIC MECHANICS OF HEALING

Healing is nothing if not a conscious act. To be effective, we need to be present. By 'present', I mean that we must be as aware as we possibly can of absolutely anything and everything that is going on inside and around us. Of course, human beings are naturally limited in this respect – under normal circumstances our minds can only give attention to, at most, two or three things at once, and even then our focus typically tends to waver quite easily.

We have (I hope) already experienced how paying gentle attention to the simple act of breathing can affect our perception of Qi. Now we're going to try to expand and deepen that perception by experimenting with posture and body mechanics, Daoist-style. Whilst much of this will be familiar to Qi Gong practitioners, it is awareness of the specific applications of body mechanics in our healing routines that might open up some relatively new territory.

As with the concept of healthy breathing, Westerners tend to have a less than an ideal grasp of what is meant by 'good posture'. Ask the average person to demonstrate good posture and they will usually stand up as straight as they can, extending the spine to its maximum, locking the knees and pinning the arms to the sides.

At the same time they will tend to puff out the chest, retract the chin and shoulder blades, and suck in the tummy. This is perfectly fine if you are in the Marines and being inspected by your colonel; otherwise, it requires a radical rethink!

The opposite end of the spectrum is even further from the ideal – namely, the round-shouldered 'slump' that sadly seems to characterize much of the population. Television, computers, poorly designed chairs and a whole host of other modern-day realities have all made their own contribution to the slump, but there is more to it than that. I would suggest that the single most damaging contributory factor in unhealthy posture is quite simply a *lack of self-awareness*, or, phrased another way, a lack of presence. As would-be healers, we need to pay more attention to this than most, not just because we wish to embody the principles of good health, but also because without a high-functioning posture it is very difficult indeed to perceive and influence Qi and to avoid energetic 'pollution'. Exactly why is this? To answer that question, let's have yet another look at some of the functional aspects of anatomy, both structural and energetic.

On the Western anatomical model, it's extremely easy to see how optimum posture might have some bearing on optimum health. The slumped stance tends to collapse the chest, radically decreasing the lungs' ability to expand and contract, and locking the diaphragm in place so that abdominal breathing is barely even an option. (In Chapter 2 we identified several good reasons why this particular scenario might best be avoided.) Meanwhile, internal organs are compressed and digestion and blood circulation compromised. The back also tends to suffer, producing chronic soft tissue tension and, if the posture is habitual, noticeable long-term deterioration of the spine, which may sometimes be irreversible. Western psychologists have also studied how posture determines state of mind – a slumped posture tends to induce a depressive state of mind, and vice versa, in a mutually dependent negative feedback loop.

Unfortunately, the ultra-upright 'marine on parade' posture is not markedly better either. Again, the diaphragm is impeded, this time by the over-rounding of the front of the thorax, and breathing tends to be restricted to the upper chest with a consequently diminished flow of oxygen. (I have actually seen extremely fit and tough British Grenadier Guards faint after about 15 minutes of trying to maintain this unnatural posture.) The entire stance is tight, strained and, not surprisingly, unsustainable. Psychologically, it promotes tension. None of this, as they say, is rocket science, but, right now, why not just allow yourself a few minutes to play with both the slumped and 'marine' ways of holding yourself. Do this sitting, standing, or preferably both.

Subtle anatomy

Anatomy in the traditional Chinese sense also includes the 'energetic anatomy'. This is where a detailed consideration of structural alignments suddenly becomes infinitely more interesting and profound.

Perhaps the first thing to say is that, *within a human being, the movement of Qi is largely NOT due to the meridian system.* Practitioners of the Daoist internal arts have long recognized that in fact most Qi within our bodies flows through (a) the body fluids, especially blood and cerebral spinal fluid, and (b) the fascia, or 'wrappings' of the soft tissue. However, as healers we must be more concerned with the meridian system itself. The principal reason for this is purely pragmatic: movement of Qi via body fluids and the fascia requires movement of the body. As QSH healers, we will be spending most of our time either standing or sitting in relatively stationary postures, working with a stationary client.

Meridian theory in QSH is more or less in accord with the energetic anatomy as seen from a Nei Gong perspective. This imposes a sort of three-part hierarchy, which is a working compromise, as the entire meridian system is clearly a single, integrated web of pathways connecting all aspects of the body-mind. However, despite this, for practical purposes it is highly useful to break it down into three constituent parts or 'layers'.

The first 'layer' of this hierarchy is the 12-meridian system that is familiar to all of us. Often these channels are referred to as the 'acquired' or 'medical' meridians. These are the ones that appear in just about every standard Acupuncture or Shiatsu textbook, and the ones that provide us with the vast majority of acupoints. (I say 'vast majority' because the acupoints along the Ren and Du Mai do not belong to this system, and obviously nor do the 'extra' points that are non-meridianal.) The reason for this apparent dominance of the 12 meridians in our thinking should be obvious: they are the ones that provide us with most of the acupoints, predictable locations through which we can gain direct entry into the energetic system.

However, in terms of how the energetic body as a whole functions, the 12-meridian system is arguably the *least important* of our three layers. Oddly enough, this comes as something of a surprise to many practitioners. It is what we could call the 'deeper energetic anatomy' that is of far more significance to us in QSH.

Deeper flows

'Deeper energetic anatomy' introduces the second layer of our energetic being, the eight 'extraordinary' or 'congenital' meridians. It is these that give us, quite literally, the blueprint around which the flesh and bones of our three-dimensional body takes shape. There are fascinating parallels between this ancient Chinese concept and the modern understanding of how cell division and growth occurs in a human foetus. Essentially, the first cell division in a fertilized ovum is in the vertical, two-dimensional plane (compatible with Chong Mai, 'Penetrating Vessel'). Next comes an 'encircling' or three-dimensional division that begins to round out the foetal shape (the oval formed by the combined Ren and Du Mai ('Conception Vessel' and 'Governing Vessel'), plus the horizontal 'belt' of Dai

Mai, 'Girdle Vessel'). After that, more complex structures begin to be made, and the tiny 'buds' of arms and legs also appear (Yin and Yang Wei Mai and Yin and Yang Qiao Mai, 'Yin and Yang Linking Vessels' and 'Yin and Yang Heel Vessels').

By contrast, the 12-meridian system is not fundamental to our basic structure. What's more, this system is still in a relatively unfinished state in a newborn baby, not reaching full development until later in childhood. This is what gives us the term 'acquired' meridian.

With the exceptions of the Ren and Du Mai, the congenital meridians do not possess their own acupoints, but instead emerge at a relatively few points 'borrowed' from along the 12 meridians. For instance, Chong Mai can be accessed via Gong Sun (SP 4) and Nei Guan (PC 6).

Structural blueprint notwithstanding, it is the energetic uses of the congenital system that really set it apart.

Daoists have employed water as a metaphor for Qi for millennia, and the image is a useful one. So, if the 12-meridian system and its collaterals can be seen metaphorically as a kind of energetic irrigation system that distributes Qi information via springs, rivulets, streams, rivers and so forth, then we must look at the congenital meridians as being more like a system of deep internal reservoirs. During a QSH session, it is often the congenital meridians that we tend to experience most powerfully.

The 'trinity'

Finally, we come to the third layer of our hierarchical model of the energetic anatomy: the trinity of the Central, Left and Right Meridians, the very core of the body's energetic being.

There has been a centuries-old debate amongst Daoist masters regarding the exact routes of the trinity. Is the Central Meridian perhaps just another name for Chong Mai? After all, the general physical location seems to correspond very well indeed. Surprisingly, some masters have answered 'yes' and some 'no' to this, and the same goes for the Left and Right Meridians with respect to the deep pathways of the Yin and Yang Qiao Mai. It seems to me that the Central Meridian is more or less identical with the Indian Yogic concept of the Sushumna Nadi, whilst the Left and Right Meridians correspond very well to the Ida and Pingala Nadis.[1]

In the most basic terms, both Indian and Chinese systems see the entire human structure as being built around a central vertical axis, uniting the perineum with the crown of the head. Furthermore, along this axis lie crucial energy centres – the three Dan Tien in the Chinese approach, or the Seven Chakras to the yogis. A debate around whether or not a Chakra is a Dan Tien would be fascinating, but is not necessary for our purposes here. Suffice to say, these vital energetic structures are all described as being 'attached' or having a 'root' on the Central Meridian or Sushumna Nadi.

In terms of location, just about everyone seems to agree that the Central Meridian is identified with the spine. Again, there is disagreement as to whether it travels inside or just in front of the spine, or, indeed, whether or not it does both of those things by splitting itself into two distinct parts – one within the marrow of the spine itself, whilst another, much more direct route connects the perineum and crown of the head in a straight line. Both pathways are envisaged as beginning at acupoint Hui Yin (CV 1) and terminating at Bai Hui (GV 20). The 'straight line' approach is generally the most useful in Qi Gong, but in QSH such concepts don't really matter. What counts is where you *feel* this energy. Meanwhile, on either side of the Central Meridian and intimately connected to it lie the Left and Right Meridians. Again, these are usually pictured as more or less straight vertical lines. I do wonder if this, too, is simply a kind of shorthand to make accessing and using these meridians a little easier? The Indian system has the Ida and Pingala Nadis criss-crossing the central axis at every Chakra, and my feeling is that this is probably structurally correct, whilst the Chinese rendition is simply functionally more expedient.

Energy gates

Energy gates (Qi Men) can sometimes be felt during a QSH session. These are sometimes mistakenly thought of as acupoints, but are actually quite different. Qi Men are step-up/step-down transformers and energy 'pumps', almost like tiny Dan Tien. They are widespread, especially at joints, although some are found deep in the interior of the body, such as in the brain. Dysfunction at Qi Men can sometimes be perceived and unblocked using QSH techniques.

One other important aspect of the energetic anatomy – the human aura – will be considered in more detail later in the book. For now, though, we have enough to begin to link the energetic structure with those aspects of refined posture that will enhance our healing abilities. What follows may well be familiar to the majority of Qi Gong or Nei Gong practitioners, but perhaps not to a good many therapists. We're also going to round the chapter off with a rather enjoyable two-person exercise that helps to put theory into practice.

The Daoists, great experimenters as ever, wished to know what was the single most useful posture for a human being to adopt. By 'useful', we mean the physical posture that will allow Qi to flow in the most unimpeded manner possible. This is the entire purpose here: to *maximize the flow of Qi*. We want to do this for several reasons, most of which should be obvious:

1. Stagnant Qi causes depletion and disease.

2. Qi that flows, grows. In other words, one important way to acquire more Qi is simply to open up our bodies to the natural movement of energy.

3. To be able to produce a healing resonance within a patient's Qi, we must have an abundance of Qi of our own. This does not mean that we are transmitting some of our Qi, however.

4. An open body posture means that we will be relatively unlikely to acquire toxic Qi from a patient. It will simply move through us and out. We need to protect ourselves from this possibility at all times.

5. Points 1–4 above are true largely by virtue of the meridian system, at least when the body is relatively static. An open posture necessarily entails an opening of the body's meridians.

Now let's look at the body mechanics of the optimum posture itself.

Exercise 3.1: Stand up!

First of all, let's look at what you're wearing. Clothing must be relatively loose, warm and comfortable. I often wear a shirt and tie to work, but even so I make sure nothing is tight enough to impede either my breathing or my stance. Footwear is important too. Make sure you have natural soles, not plastic or rubber. To enhance Qi flow you need excellent contact with the ground, and so obviously 'fashion footwear' is out. These days I opt for comfortable, leather-soled men's shoes.

Stand with your feet roughly shoulder-width apart. The exact distance between the feet varies from individual to individual, due to slightly different shoulder- to hip-width ratios.

Experiment until you find your own ideal width. It will be the one that feels most 'right' to you.

Now ensure that your feet are parallel: this means the outside edge of both feet should be parallel with each other, whilst you should also be able to draw a straight line connecting the tips of the toes of each foot (see Figure 3.1).

Ensure that your body weight is slightly forward, that there is more weight on the ball of the foot than on the heel. This allows a splaying of the bones at the front of the foot that in turn allows the all-important Yong Quan (KD 1) acupoint to open. (Yong Quan is our vital energetic connection with Di Qi (earthly Qi). There will be more about earthly Qi in a later chapter.) Of course, this is just an 'optimum' posture. Once you feel a sensation of Qi in your feet and legs, it's perfectly permissible to walk about or adopt another stance, so long as it allows for the free-flow of Qi. The same basic principles always apply.

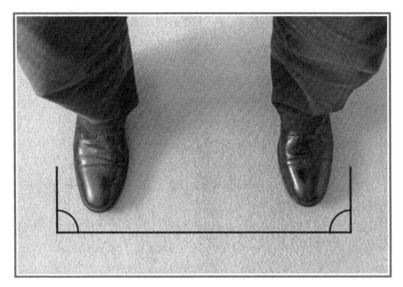

Figure 3.1: Parallel alignment of feet

Bend your knees. It doesn't have to be by very much, and if you can no longer see your toes, you have gone too far! However, there is an important Daoist internal arts maxim at play here: 'Never bone on bone.' This simply means if you straighten a joint to its full extension (until the bones touch), you will cut off the free-flow of Qi. This rule goes for every single joint in your body. Always try to create a slight curve, bend or gap in a joint, however subtle.

Straighten the spine. This statement needs some qualification. Remember the upright marine? That is not what we want here at all. By a straight spine, the Daoists meant one wherein the vertebrae were very slightly teased apart. The ancient metaphor for this was to see the spine as the supple string of a necklace, with each vertebra acting as one of the necklace's pearls. These 'pearls' should be very gently separated, but absolutely without strain. This arrangement makes a considerable difference to Qi flow in the Central Meridian and Du Mai.

Imagine that you are being gently suspended from the acupoint Bai Hui (GV 20) at the vertex of the skull. Traditionally, one envisaged a golden thread connecting this point to the heavens. Qi Gong master Kenneth Cohen recommends instead that you see yourself hanging from a 'sky hook'. Do whatever works for you, but try to be constantly aware of the need to let your skull float free of the top of the neck, even if by only a millimetre.

Once you have mastered this erect, but relaxed, posture, start to allow all the flesh of your body to 'melt' downwards under the influence of gravity. In Qi Gong circles this process is known as 'sinking and relaxing'. However, do not relax so much that your skeletal structure becomes compromised.

Make sure that there is always some space in your armpit area, and that your arms are not touching the sides of the body.

Allow your feet to 'sink' into the ground. This is as much a mental process as a physical one. At the same time, try to allow a sinking around the joint at the front of the foot, approximately around acupoint Jie Xi (ST 41). Meanwhile try to extend upwards around the Achilles tendon, possibly around Fu Liu (KD 7). These movements are very subtle and hard to master. If you can't do them, don't worry; they come with practice.

Again, it is principally the mind and a firm intention to relax these parts of the body that will get you the results you want. In general, sinking at the front of the body whilst raising up at the back allows for greater movement of Qi, especially in the Ren and Du Mai.

Place the tip of your tongue gently against the roof of your mouth. This helps to open the Central Meridian.

Breathe gently from your lower abdomen, allowing the ribs to move out laterally and the lower back to expand too. If this does not work for you at first, just relax. The main thing is never to force it.

You should now be standing, perfectly comfortably, in the optimum Daoist internal arts stance, meridians as open as possible and mind calm but focused. This is also the optimum QSH stance. Compare yourself with Figure 3.2 to see how you're doing. A mirror can help, but another person's opinion is even better in this case.

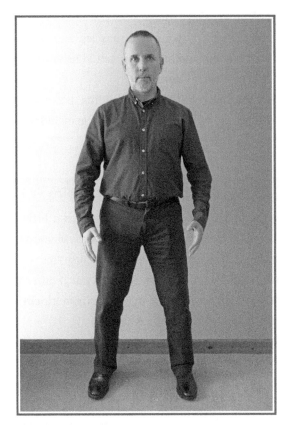

Figure 3.2: Basic standing posture

Exercise 3.2: Sit down!

At least 50 per cent of the healing I undertake is from a sitting position. This is basically just an adaptation of the standing posture, and was created by the Daoists for much the same reason: to maximize Qi flow.

Select a good chair for this, one which is not too squashy and neither too high nor too low. In terms of height, the perfect chair is one that allows you to have your feet flat on the floor, with a 90-degree bend at the knees. (Obviously gravity isn't working on our feet in quite the same way here as when we stand, and *as long as contact with the floor is maintained at all times*, we don't need to worry too much about putting most of our weight on the front of the foot.) Sit forward, so that your spine is supported by your own muscles, and not by the chair. Otherwise, your posture and breathing should be exactly the same as for the standing posture in Exercise 3.1.

Practise until both seated and standing postures become an integrated and 'everyday' aspect of your muscle memory.

Exercise 3.3: The test of a good posture

If everything that we've discussed above seems a little formal, it's now time to have some serious fun. It's fun because you are invited to clown around with a partner, and serious because this is a very direct way to prove to oneself and others just how much difference correct or incorrect body alignments can make to our meridian system. It's also very easy.

Stand in the healing posture detailed above, as in Exercise 3.1. Allow yourself to be comfortable and relaxed.

Ask a partner to stand at 90 degrees to you, but within arm's length.

When you're both ready, your partner is going to push steadily against your shoulder. You will try to resist (see Figure 3.3). (Please note: this isn't a pushing contest! The person standing at the side will always tend to win, but the purpose here is simply to prove that the push can be resisted for a few moments before structure is compromised and the feet are obliged to move.)

Now perform exactly the same exercise, but make sure that your arms are firmly clamped against your sides. Try to resist the push – you can't! You should find that you are easily toppled and have very little power to resist. Why? Because clamping your arms to your sides shuts down the Left and Right Meridians, with a subsequent loss of Qi flow.

Now try again, but this time lock your knees instead of clamping the arms. The same thing should happen. The body's natural 'Qi structure' has been hampered, and you are the weaker for it.

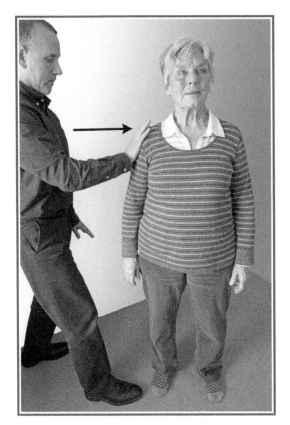

Figure 3.3: Shoulder push

This is an admittedly crude but graphic demonstration of just how important maintaining correct bodily alignment really is. As a QSH healer, you need to take this aspect of the discipline very seriously indeed. Your Qi needs to flow unimpeded if you are to help others, and avoid becoming sick yourself.

Notes

1. A Nadi is a conduit for Prana, the Indian correlate for Qi, and is usually described as a 'subtle tube' – in other words, a meridian.

Chapter 4

INTENTION IS EVERYTHING

In this chapter we are going to investigate another key element of QSH: the vital role played by *intention*.

Earlier in the book I talked about what I choose to call *noticing*, which can be seen as a direct result of how present we are able and willing to be at any given moment. The ability to notice, to be absolutely present, is essential in QSH. However, without firm intention, presence is almost unachievable – there's no attention without intention.

First of all, then, to define intention we need to understand the role of willpower, or Zhi. Zhi differs slightly from the Western concept of the will, in that it is absolutely *not* a fixed attribute of an individual. The strength and therefore the usefulness of Zhi does not stem from any innate, immutable personal characteristic, but rather from an expression of that person's energetic health at any given moment. In other words, it can and does change, depending on circumstances.

Zhi is intimately related to the Chinese concept of the Kidney, and is therefore ultimately rooted in Jing, our most fundamental raw form of energy. It is also dependent on the integrity of 'Minister

Fire', the motivating force provided by the Ming Men traditionally located between the kidneys and also inextricably linked, amongst other things, with the mobilization of Jing. It follows therefore that a healthy mind really does require a healthy body. Mind and body are inseparable and inter-dependent. In our practice we need to embody the principle to make it real. We need to be as healthy as we possibly can.

What, then, of my premise that there can be no attention without intention? It is a carefully cultivated Zhi that provides a level of intention that can be sustained for long periods.

Important though it undoubtedly is, however, Zhi is certainly not the sole component required in the creation of prolonged periods of awareness. We must also cultivate the quality of Yi, the 'spirit' of the Spleen organ system. Yi can be defined as something approaching the Western concept of 'cognitive aptitude', our ability to think. Although QSH often deliberately bypasses thinking altogether, we nevertheless require a strong Yi to enable clarity to manifest. Without it, everything becomes muzzy. Again, Yi is highly dependent on a strong supply of Qi for its robustness, this time from the Spleen Meridian system. It is unlikely, however, that you will ever meet a person who possesses a strong Spleen coupled with weak Kidney energy. Viewed this way, Zhi is the foundation stone that supports the perceptive abilities of Yi.

The 'monkey mind'

Human beings are in one sense 'thinking machines', and have a strong bias towards interpreting the world via the medium of our thoughts. We like to categorize, to name things.

Our minds insist on providing endless running commentaries and are all too easily seduced into going off at a tangent. This is what the Daoists call the 'monkey mind'. Needless to say, this is pretty much the diametric opposite of what we are aiming for in a QSH healing session.

In Qi Gong circles there is an aphorism that it is absolutely crucial for any healer to understand and to be able to put into practice: 'Yi Dao, Qi Dao'. This compact traditional phrase translates as something like 'where the intention leads, the Qi must inevitably follow' or 'where the mind goes, energy flows'. Let us depart from theory for a few moments and see if we can begin to develop a more physically rooted, visceral feel for the notion of Yi Dao, Qi Dao.

In this exercise we are going to begin to sharpen up our natural ability to tell the difference between directed attention and its opposite – mere daydreaming!

Exercise 4.1: Bringing the mind to the hands

Stand, or sit, in the open, receptive posture described earlier in this book (see Exercise 3.1).

Clasp your hands gently together. There is no need to squeeze or apply pressure – it's best that you don't.

Close your eyes, and focus as clearly as you can on your breathing for a few moments.

Once your breathing seems calm and your mind reasonably present, bring your attention back to your clasped hands.

Feel the connection between your hands. Notice where skin touches skin. Be aware of the bones, the joints. Now mentally take note of any warmth, cold, stiffness, tension or, for that matter, relaxation in the hands. Can you feel tingling, electricity? Something that might even be Qi? Can you feel the blood pulsing? Is that in any way distinct from any more subtle pulsing you might also be experiencing? There is no right answer here, only awareness of what *is*.

Do your hands feel somehow 'different' simply because you are focusing on them in this way? (We don't need to define 'different' here: any sensation is valid, however crude or rarefied it might be.) All that is required of you right now is to notice anything and everything that is arising, if possible without judgement or internal comment. On the other hand, if your mind is giving a blow-by-blow account of every moment you are experiencing, don't get tense. Minds do that! Just don't take yourself too seriously, and keep trying to focus as best you can.

Now, once you have some sense of the relative levels of 'aliveness' in your hands, you can begin to make use of your Zhi and Yi to manipulate your experience. Without generating any internal tension, gently 'ask' your Qi to start flowing from your right hand into your left.

Don't tense your hands whilst doing this! It is also good to try to exercise a little respectful humility here – the Qi does not need you to give it commands!

What are you feeling now? Can you feel any kind of flow occurring from right to left? Has the volume and quality of sensation in the hands changed at all? Is there any sense of something 'travelling' up your left forearm? The specifics do not matter, but really do try to notice whatever happens, log it in your mind, and, at the same time, try not to think any more about it or analyse it in any way. To the best of your ability, be the passive observer.

After a minute or two, reverse the flow. Now your mind is requesting Qi to flow from the left hand into the right. Again, simply notice what happens in as much detail as you can. Is this the same experience as previously, or slightly different? Continue for a little while, until you are satisfied that you have felt everything that you can. Finally, unclasp your hands and give them a little shake out.

As I have noted above, we are, to a great extent, thinking machines. So how do we stop thinking for long enough to do our job well? We practise, practise, practise. Then we let go of trying to control our thoughts and our environment, and just trust that we have trained ourselves well enough to be effective as a healer. A sense of humour helps... If we drift, we drift (and we will!). The task is to notice ourselves doing this and to return to a state of presence, of relaxed awareness. It doesn't matter if we have to do this a hundred times or a thousand times during a healing session. What matters is that we do it.

Eventually, we may find that we have gained a certain mastery, and that the duration of our periods of non-attention and daydreaming has become less and less. Basically, this is meditation. It does not take any special human ability to do this. All it takes is a reasonably high level of health and a great deal of persistence. Another word that could be substituted here instead of persistence is, of course, willpower – yet another application of Zhi.

Before presenting you with another, slightly more challenging training exercise, I'd like to round off this chapter with a brief discussion of one more inherent difference between QSH and External Qi Healing (EQH) – the principal hands-on healing paradigm on offer in modern Chinese hospitals. Appropriately, this is with reference to our understanding of the word 'intention'.

Two very different approaches

As discussed in the Introduction to this book, EQH is a branch of Traditional Chinese Medicine (TCM), the style of state-sanctioned – some would say regimented – medical care that became dominant in China after the Communist revolution of the 20th century. Here in the West, TCM has its advocates and detractors. I myself find it highly useful as an acupuncturist, and use it extensively alongside other styles in the clinic. I even have some training in EQH and use that too, from time to time. However, despite both being rooted in and inspired by the Chinese Medicine of antiquity, TCM's EQH and QSH bear only the most superficial resemblance to each other. Please note that this is in no way a discussion of which system is 'best' or even of which could lay claim to any authenticity. (Some would say neither! QSH is obviously something I myself put together from Daoist inspirations, and some critics even view TCM as a greatly simplified interpretation of ancient practices.)

In EQH, 'intention' is used in two distinct ways: (1) to assess the state of the client's Qi, as interpreted in the familiar 'pattern differentiation' style of TCM. This leads to diagnosis and a treatment plan; (2) to project Qi from the healer into the client, often via acupoints. Many specific techniques are used for this, depending on the healer's assessment. A typical example would be 'Swordfinger', a hand posture that allows for a concentrated beam of Qi to pass from the therapist into the client. The therapist is very much 'in control', skilfully manipulating the client's Qi in direct accordance with a TCM diagnosis that has already been arrived at. Sometimes the opposite is also true: EQH healers may 'pull out' or 'dredge' excess or stagnant Qi from a client's system. Even so, this is still a highly directed, therapist-controlled approach.

By contrast, in QSH, intention is indeed used to determine both the quality and quantity of Qi in a client, but no clinical diagnosis follows as a result. Whatever is there is acutely felt but not analysed by the intellect. It is what it is, no labelling necessary. The treatment that follows is intuition-based, not prescriptive, with the therapist's hands simply 'knowing' what to do, and the therapist's mind passively observing the process. QSH is therefore substantially less analytical than EQH. By the time you have finished reading this book, you will have been provided with all the tools you need to arrive at a high level of intuitive understanding of your client's Qi, and you will also just 'know' what to do.

There is a second, and equally important, distinction between EQH and QSH. *QSH does not in any way require the therapist to project Qi.* Instead, the therapist's intention is very clearly geared towards merely experiencing the client's Qi. Any manipulation or directing of the Qi is carried out via a gentle mental bias, giving 'encouragement' to the Qi to re-set and re-balance itself into that state of ever greater coherence that we call 'health'. To achieve the result we want, all that is required is to be vividly present.

Awareness is everything, although yes, we will sometimes be using subtle movements of the hands to encourage the Qi to flow. However, there is no directed 'searchlight beam' of Qi being used here, no projection. In this respect, QSH is demonstrably far more passive (perhaps 'meditative' would be a more accurate word) than EQH.

Let us now try to get a greater feel for this meditative, 'watching' quality of QSH. It's time for another exercise. This one requires a partner and, preferably, a treatment couch. An ordinary bed or sofa can often be pressed into service if nothing else is available.

Exercise 4.2: An unmediated experience of Qi

Ask your partner to lie down comfortably on the treatment couch, facing upwards. Use whatever pillows, blankets, etc. might seem appropriate – this procedure might take some time!

Sit closely behind your partner and cradle the back of their head in your hands. Ideally, on each side, several of your fingers should be approximately touching the location of acupoints Tian Zhu (UB 10) and Feng Chi (GB 20) on the back of the neck, as in Figure 4.1.

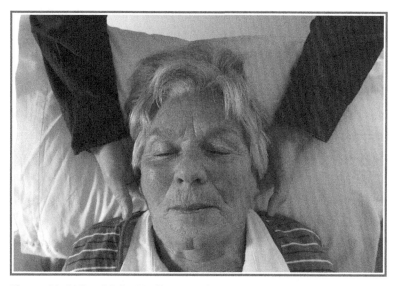

Figure 4.1: Qi Sensitivity Healing practice

It is useful to be fairly precise with point location here, although in practice it's usually fine to be within half a centimetre or so of an acupoint. In any case, holding the skull like this means that you'll be covering quite a few acupoints anyway. (Therapists will probably already know a great deal about the functions of individual acupoints

– for instance, that Feng Chi subdues Liver Yang, expels Pathogenic Wind, etc. *For the purposes of all the exercises in this book, I'd like you to set that knowledge aside completely, at least for now.*)

Point location notwithstanding, we are aiming for an unmediated experience of Qi, and so our accumulated knowledge and concepts can only hinder us. Get your mind out of the way! If you find this approach a little too iconoclastic for your tastes, please remember that it is a quintessentially Daoist approach!

Try not to talk at this stage. Instead, concentrate on your breathing, as described in Chapter 2. You are aiming for a meditative mood here. Try, too, to be aware of your partner's breathing, if possible without drawing conclusions about it. You should aim to be every bit as aware of your partner as you are of yourself, as each impression you have of them helps build up your 'intuitive picture' of their energetic status. Avoid intellectualizing if you possibly can.

Breathe in this rather empty-minded way for at least a minute or two. Undoubtedly, your thoughts will wander, but this isn't a problem as long as you constantly chivvy them back to the task in hand. Be gentle with yourself as you do this. It's all too easy to get into the self-critical mindset of 'Oh, my mind is so stupid. I can't do this. I just can't focus today', and so forth. If this happens, be amused at yourself, rather than frustrated. It helps.

Now, when you're ready, bring your attention back to where your hands and fingers lie on your partner's head and neck.

What do you feel? Become fascinated by the texture of skin, the muscles and tendons, the feel of the underlying skeletal structure. Is there tension in your partner's neck? Is there warmth, moisture, a feeling of 'aliveness'? Can you feel the blood pulsing? Perceive everything you possibly can, but do not allow yourself to analyse exactly what it is that you are feeling.

Can you detect the difference between the sensations in your partner's body and those in your own? Can you tell which pulsing of the blood is theirs and which is yours?

Finally, can you feel something that is 'other'? Not the blood, not random nerve impulses in your own hands, but a distinct presence of something indefinable but very, very alive. Could this be Qi? What is it like? Warm, perhaps? Fluid, tingling, stagnant, healthy, sick? Is it light or heavy? Ethereal or sludge-like?

Do the Qi sensations change under your hands as you become aware of them? In the most general sense, how vital, or otherwise, does the Qi feel?

Does this experience of Qi strike you as somehow different in the vicinity of acupoints than in ordinary body tissues? Is a subtle, but increasingly obvious, 'pulsing' of this Qi sensation beginning to build, especially at the acupoints? (It is important that you are able to notice here the qualitative differences between your own Qi and that of the person you are working with. This can take practice. In the main, it just requires paying attention.)

Wait until you feel this energetic pulsing (quite distinct from the pulsing of blood) becoming so strong that you simply can't ignore it. Does the sense of 'dynamic aliveness' in your partner suddenly seem more vivid to you?

Experience how your partner's head, neck, breathing and general state of relaxation are right now, in this moment. Has anything changed? What exactly? Stop thinking; keep feeling.

Keep going for a few more minutes.

Even though you have in one sense done absolutely nothing at all, does it nevertheless feel as if an *interaction* of some kind has taken place, one that has mysteriously changed the quality of your partner's energy?

Return to your breathing, and when you're ready, gently disengage. Make sure that your partner is fine, and then go and have a cup of tea.

No doubt you were absent numerous times during this exploration. Perhaps, too, if you're absolutely honest, you may have felt very little during the interaction and did not perceive anything that could reasonably be called Qi. Some people don't experience much at first, and that is perfectly acceptable for now. The skills you require will come with practice, and if you are prepared to engage with them, you are already well on your way to becoming a QSH healer.

Chapter 5

HANDS OFF!

So far we have only looked at QSH in the context of a 'hands-on' modality, where touching or holding the patient in various ways can bring about the result we seek.

Perhaps surprisingly, this represents less than half of the QSH approach. In this chapter we will be deepening our awareness of Qi considerably by looking at what happens *outside* the body when attention is brought to bear. In other words, we're going to engage in some 'hands-off' work.

Ancient peoples around the world had an almost universal understanding that not only the human body but also, indeed, the physical structure of absolutely anything that could be said to be alive did not in any way demarcate the outer limits of the energy body. They perceived that we extend beyond our flesh-and-bone packaging in a very real, palpable way. I am speaking here, of course, about the so-called 'aura'. Unfortunately, the concept of the aura has often been either sensationalized or obfuscated, attracting far more mystical interpretations than it really requires.

The Daoists recognized the aura quite simply as a seamless, natural extension of the human energy field. As usual, they devoted a great deal of time and attention to exploring this aspect of a human being, and have thus been able to hand down to us a detailed, functional and predictably practical understanding. Because the word 'aura' has become so laden with meanings that are not helpful to us with regard to QSH, I have decided instead to refer to it by the somewhat less emotive term 'extended energy field' (EEF).

As with any other aspect of Qi, the ancient peoples understood that the EEF could be worked with, balanced and healed. In QSH, dealing with these energies represents a substantial portion of what we should be aiming to do. The ability to *see* and elaborate on visual information from the EEF is highly coveted in many New Age circles, and I have met quite a few people who claim to have this talent. I think it's worth stating here that most of us simply do not seem to have it. I certainly don't, and therefore I have never tried to apply it to my work in the clinic. Fortunately, one does not have to. In QSH, being able to see the EEF is pretty much irrelevant. Being able to *feel* the complexities, subtleties and dysfunctions of the EEF, however, is an absolutely crucial skill. For most of us, this is a much more achievable and, I believe, useful ability than aura reading.

So let's try to experience what a person's EEF actually feels like. Once again, you will need a partner for this.

Exercise 5.1: Working with another person's EEF

Ask your partner to stand in a relaxed way, with their back to you. They do not have to adopt the stance recommended by QSH, but do at least try to make sure that their knees have a small amount of bend in them, for reasons which by now should be obvious to you.

Suggest to your partner that they might want to 'go with' whatever happens, but otherwise give no intimation of what you are intending to do. People can be extremely suggestible. If you set up an expectation for what a person might experience, that inevitably tends to colour what they actually do experience.

So, standing behind your partner (where they can't see you and so are not influenced by your movements), extend your hands with the palms facing their mid-to-upper back, as shown in Figure 5.1. The distance you stand from them will vary depending on who you are working with, but roughly one metre away is usually about right. As ever, take a few moments to concentrate on your own breathing. Let everything settle and become quiet.

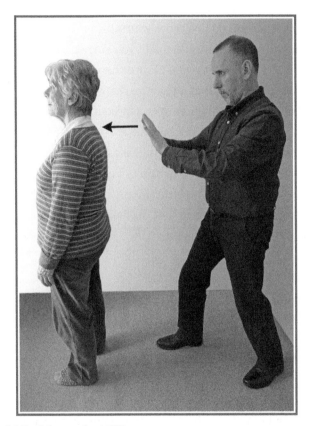

Figure 5.1: Pushing against EEF

Now try to feel the edge of your partner's EEF by gently reaching out towards them with both palms simultaneously. (Don't over-extend your arms. Be relaxed about this.) You may need to shuffle forward or backward a little until you find the optimum spot.

Can you perceive a non-visible 'border', at which you start to encounter your partner's EEF? What does it feel like? Does the air suddenly feel more dense, or perhaps more alive at this border? (It's fine to close your eyes if that helps you to focus your mind on what your hands are experiencing.)

What is the sensation in your hands? Does the edge of the EEF feel vibrant? Is your subjective impression of it one of health or of disharmony? Is it light or sluggish? Is it warm or cold, tingly or stagnant?

Slowly explore the edge of the EEF with your hands. Be totally honest with yourself: do not allow yourself to imagine that you are feeling particular sensations if actually you are not.

Assuming you can feel the EEF, are there any aspects to it that you are intuitively drawn to, or that perhaps feel somehow 'wrong' to you? Are there places where you unaccountably want to linger? Do you have any urge to 'smooth out' or pull at any parts of the EEF? Do you feel as if you could extrude it as if it were something you could literally stretch and compress, like chewing gum? Don't analyse or label any of this, and, for now, don't try to do anything specific with the EEF or attempt to perform any healing on it. What we're doing now is really just a demonstration.

Allow your hands to rove around the edges of the EEF as if they had a will of their own.

Once again, this is really just a matter of getting your mind, your agenda and, frankly, your ego, out of the way.

Now, begin slowly and rhythmically to 'push' against your partner's EEF. No physical strength should be applied here, and nor should you be exerting any mental force. Instead, your intent should be clear and focused, but perfectly relaxed.

At the end of each push, slowly draw your palms back towards you whilst still focusing on the EEF. Does it seem to follow you at all, to stick to your hands? Does it ebb and flow with your movements?

Keep this up for a little while and notice if your partner starts to 'rock' backwards and forwards in perfect time with your actions, as if they were somehow being gently pushed and pulled by an invisible magnet.

Keep going. Notice if this swaying or rocking motion gets more and more obvious. (Remember that your partner can't see what you are doing. It's important that they don't take visual cues from you.)

Stop when you feel you have done enough. As often as not, it is actually your partner who will put a stop to proceedings, simply because otherwise they might topple over! I have several times managed to induce such a swaying motion in a partner that they literally fell over backwards and had to be caught! Just be aware that this really can happen.

It might be fun at this point to reverse roles – let your partner take over and see if they can latch on to your EEF in such a way that you perceive the connection and then be physically moved. Remember: don't fool yourself into believing that something is happening if it's not.

Try not to predict or pre-empt anything at all. You have nothing to prove.

The structure and functions of the extended energy field

It is difficult to think of any ancient wisdom tradition that did not embrace the concept of the EEF. Highly specific references to it can be found in Native American, Australian Aboriginal, African, Tibetan, Chinese and Indian sources, and this list is by no means exhaustive. Perhaps the halo surrounding the heads of Christian saints is just another expression of the EEF, and in Islam the Sufis appear to be aware of energy fields too. As I have noted earlier, the aura is also one of the cornerstones of many New Age practices, although in such cases descriptions usually tally broadly with the Indian yogic understanding.

Any differences in how the EEF was understood can perhaps be ascribed to cultural leanings. Again, we tend to perceive what we are expecting to perceive.

The following is an example taken from the Inka tradition of Peru, championed in the West principally by anthropologist-cum-shaman Alberto Villoldo. Here is part of Villoldo's description of the EEF, as conceived by the Inka: 'Imagine you are enveloped in a translucent, multicoloured orb pulsing with blues, greens, magentas and yellows, enfolding you to the width of your outstretched arms' (2001, p.43).

(Interestingly, the Inka also seemed to have had a detailed knowledge of what appears to be the meridian system, called by them 'rios de luz', or 'rivers of light'. Chakras, or possibly the three Dan Tien, known as 'pukios', 'wells of light', are also both recognized and heavily used in this system. Inka healing was to a great extent concerned with perceiving and releasing malignant energetic formations within the EEF.)

The huge body of yogic literature from ancient India often goes into remarkable detail about the EEF. Again, a 'cocoon' of subtle energy is conceived as surrounding the body, intimately connected to the Chakras. In this Indian system (as with several others), the EEF is purported to incorporate different 'layers' of energy within its structure, each of which vibrates within a particular frequency band, and therefore also manifests its own identifying colour. The frequency bands are to be thought of as containing increasingly subtle energetic vibrations, the most ethereal being of an almost purely spiritual nature. Each of these layers is given a name (causal, etheric,[1] etc.), and each is also credited with its own highly specific function – some of them animate and protect the physical body whilst others provide us with our emotional, intellectual and spiritual capacities. There are said to be seven of these layers (corresponding to the Indian idea of Seven Chakras). Other traditions sometimes identify a different number of layers, four being common. In most systems, each of these layers of the aura are conceived of as emanating from the spine or from an equivalent of the Central Meridian, as if they were nested one inside another, like Russian dolls. Again, different people have viewed things in their own way, and therefore I feel it is important not to become too engaged in championing one system over another. This is not in any way to suggest that 'anything goes', but simply that all these different ways of regarding the EEF can have great validity when used in the cultural context they were intended for.

So what of the Chinese? What is their (inevitably Daoist) concept of the EEF?

I think it fair to say that the Daoist system is on the whole a little less concerned with the EEF than are many of the world's other wisdom traditions (although it is true that some modern Qi Gong healers use aura colour differentiation for diagnosis and treatment).

Generally, the congenital and acquired meridian systems and the three Dan Tien seem always to have been more of a focus. Despite this, the Daoists did, of course, explore the EEF in some detail, and this is largely the conceptual model that I use in QSH.

As in the systems outlined briefly above, the Daoists conceive of the EEF as a 'bubble' of energy surrounding the body. It is roughly egg-shaped, slightly more pointed at the top and rounded below, and extends approximately one metre beyond the physical body in the average healthy adult. (Note that this means the EEF extends down into the ground. This will become important in a later chapter.) Again, the EEF is regarded as a kind of energetic storehouse of 'information', rather like the hard drive in a computer. In a similar way to a computer, the nature of the information stored is binary – in other words, it operates through the interplay of Yin and Yang energies. Much of this data trapped within the EEF refers to past traumas and significant emotional events. Specialized Daoist healing techniques, as well as breathing and meditation applications, have been created to release and harmonize this trapped, dysfunctional Qi, and, needless to say, some of these have been tremendously influential in the creation of QSH.

The extended energy field and intuition

The Daoists also regard the EEF as a kind of energetic 'antenna', in the sense of an apparatus for perceiving the Qi of other living beings, and, most especially, of other humans. This level of perception is usually below the cognitive level, and so we may only be conscious of it as sensory impressions – perhaps an unaccountable instant attraction to, or dislike of, the personality of another. Most of us have experienced this kind of otherwise inexplicable intuition. As a QSH healer, this is precisely the faculty we are seeking to harness. *Looked at in this way, intuition is revealed as no more or less than the perception of interacting energy fields.* Any individual who is prepared to be present enough to acknowledge such interactions as they occur will quickly develop a high level of intuition. Consequently, in a healing scenario, they will just 'know' what to do to benefit their client the most. Intuition can be trained.

Another aspect of the EEF that is arguably emphasized more in Daoism than any of the other traditions is the direct relationship between the field and the breath. Again, this is clinically important in QSH, as we shall see in a subsequent chapter. In essence, the EEF expands as we inhale, and contracts when we exhale. The inhalation 'supercharges' the EEF with an abundance of fresh Qi.

As for 'layers' within the EEF, Daoism is far less definite than the other systems. The Qi contained within the bubble of the EEF is regarded as fairly formless, with the exception of the defensive layer, or Wei Qi, which extends like a protective sheath just beyond the skin. The outer edges of the EEF are said to be easily perceptible, almost like a membrane, and layers of energy can sometimes be perceived, even within a patient's body. In QSH these do not need to be analysed.

In my own experience, it is indeed easy to locate the outer limits of the EEF with one's hands, although I would never describe what I find as being like a membrane. To me, it's more like the fuzzy, vibrating boundary of an energetic 'cloud', one that is constantly expanding and contracting in exact time with the breath. Layers of energetic activity can often be perceived within the field, and these can be felt to exhibit different qualities of sensation as one moves one's hands questingly, to and fro.

Exercise 5.2: Feeling the three Dan Tien

This is yet another partner exercise requiring a treatment couch. This time we're going to heighten our ability to feel and manipulate energies within the three Dan Tien. As we have already seen, these step-up/step-down transformers are major elements of the energy body as recognized in Daoism. In the clinic you will be working with them a great deal. Despite each Dan Tien having a physical location within the body, this is nevertheless a 'hands-off' exercise.

Ask your partner to lie down comfortably on the couch, face up.

Assume the appropriate stance, or, if you prefer, sit on a chair close to the couch. As discussed earlier in the book, the sitting position requires the same loose-jointed, open posture as in standing. Make sure your feet are in both in good contact with the floor. Sitting or standing, make sure your hands will easily be able to reach the three Dan Tien as you allow them to float over your partner's body.

Focus on your breathing. Let the room become very still.

Now bring one hand, palm down, to a location roughly four to six inches above your partner's lower Dan Tien. Your other hand should be a little out to one side of you, palm facing the floor (see Figure 5.2).

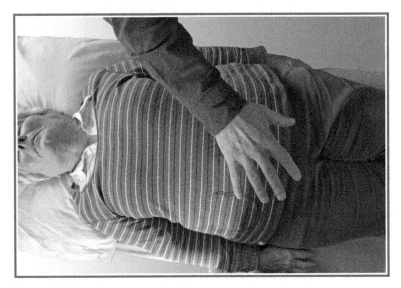

Figure 5.2: Palm hovers over Dan Tien

Keep the hand poised above the lower Dan Tien. What can you feel?

Now move the hand slowly in a clockwise direction, all the while paying close attention to what sensations you may be receiving through your palm or fingers. Keep this up for at least two minutes (see Figure 5.3).

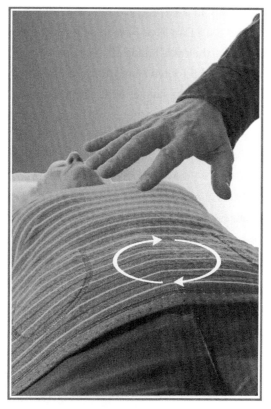

Figure 5.3: Clockwise rotation of palm

Reverse the direction of your hand to anti-clockwise. Does this make a difference to your impressions?

After a minute or two, go back to rotating your hand clockwise above the Dan Tien. Can you feel anything that wasn't there before? Maybe the air above the abdomen feels somehow thicker or more alive? Perhaps, in some strange, inexplicable way, you feel as if you are actually reaching into your partner's body and stirring the Qi in their Dan Tien, even though you are not touching them at all. (Verbal feedback is always welcome, but if your partner says they feel nothing whatsoever, don't worry. Healing is still taking place. What matters in QSH is that you, the healer, clearly perceive what is going on.)

What else do you notice about your partner right now? Is there any sense of 'letting go', of a deeper level of relaxation? Changes in breathing? Falling deeply asleep, even? Watch, but do not analyse.

Once you feel you have worked sufficiently with the lower Dan Tien, repeat the entire procedure with the middle Dan Tien in the centre of the chest, and then the upper Dan Tien, in the forehead. Mentally note any qualitative differences between the three.

How will you know when the exercise is finished? By intuition, of course!

When you are ready, bring both of your hands into your lap and return to a simple awareness of your breathing.

Notes

1. The word 'etheric' can be a cause of some confusion. Depending on one's source, it can refer to a specific layer of the EEF, or, alternatively, the term 'etheric body' can sometimes be used to mean the EEF in its entirety.

Chapter 6

GOING DEEPER

Technique versus 'feel'

It should be fairly obvious by now that the QSH system is somewhat more passive in its approach than its TCM equivalent, EQH. We have seen that QSH is firmly rooted in perceiving and observing, and does not share EQH's reliance on formal pattern differentiation. Nor is QSH based on directing, releasing and, most particularly, on transmitting Qi. Instead, the interaction between therapist and patient is largely a case of effecting change via a mutual 'meeting' of energies. This means that it is best not to view QSH as an intervention performed by one person on another. This is a matter of emphasis, because yes, sometimes we do seek to influence a person's Qi to move or re-configure in its own particular way, but this is not where our emphasis lies.

We should also bear in mind that QSH differs from other healing approaches in that it is designed to be used either on its own as a stand-alone system, or in tandem with whatever therapy you already employ. Both can be performed simultaneously, during the same session.

So, whilst you may have used considerable intellectual deduction within a recognized diagnostic framework in the treatment of your patient, the QSH 'portion' of that treatment will be largely tactile and intuitive, and therefore decidedly non-intellectual and non-diagnostic.

It is also true that QSH is far less technique-based than EQH. EQH healers spend many, many hours developing their ability to project Qi in particular ways, and have a large vocabulary of techniques at their disposal. For example, the ability to project a 'beam' of Qi that is strong enough to literally bend a candle flame as much as one metre away is highly prized in EQH. (I have actually witnessed this.) Such an undoubtedly impressive skill can take years to cultivate, and results in the capacity to direct a large amount of healing energy in a highly concentrated form into acupoints or other specific areas of a patient's body. In QSH, this is not at all what we are intending to do. As any good Daoist might tell us, technique isn't everything. *Sometimes, less really is more!*

In developing the mindset of QSH, I have consciously attempted to adapt tried-and-trusted Daoist *principles* rather than importing specific Daoist techniques. That is not to say that QSH lacks any technique at all; in fact, there are actually quite a number of 'manoeuvres' that I use which are designed to be learned, practised and perfected. (These evolved in a 'trial and error' fashion over a long period of time in the clinic, which, of course, is how most Daoist medical accomplishments came about in the first place. The physical techniques of QSH will be presented in some detail in later chapters of this book.)

We can say, then, that far from abandoning technical accomplishment altogether, QSH 'techniques' are indeed applied during a healing session. However, this is never the end result of an intellectual process based on pattern diagnosis (or, for that matter, a five-element diagnosis, hara examination or any other formal system you may already follow). Instead, it is performed at the sole bidding of intuition, and is brought to bear spontaneously in response to one's 'sub-conscious' reading of the patient's energy field at any given moment. But is this not merely an undisciplined, even random, 'do whatever takes your fancy' approach? Most certainly not! As should be clear by now, QSH requires a theoretical knowledge of the meridian system, good point location skills, a highly developed feel for Qi, as well as an almost unshakeable mental focus. Everything else issues naturally from there.

So if Daoist principles underlie the application of technique in QSH, exactly which principles? Central to our approach is that old Daoist chestnut: the concept of Wu-Wei.

Wu-Wei – the interface between action and non-action

Relatively easy to explain, Wu-Wei is often extraordinarily difficult to manifest in one's own life! QSH is in many ways my own attempt to provide a physical application for this most fascinating, elusive concept. So what is Wu-Wei?

> The Dao does nothing and yet leaves nothing undone. (Lao Tzu, *Dao De Jing*)

This famous line of Lao Tzu's comes from what is undoubtedly the most influential Daoist text of all time, and has been interpreted in various ways. We could understand it as an intimation of the mysterious, mystical nature of Dao, or we could treat it as an especially wise piece of advice on how to apply Wu-Wei in our daily existence. Seen in this light, Wu-Wei emerges as a powerful method of applying *naturalness* to our every action. Its opposite is known in Chinese as Yu-Wei, which we could translate as something like 'making an excessive effort' or 'swimming against the tide'. To tread the path of Yu-Wei is to be nothing less than un-natural.

Wu-Wei, then, really means 'going with the flow'. This does not in any sense imply fatalism, laziness or a refusal to take responsibility for our actions. One can only go with the flow of events if one has a clear perception of what that flow is. This implies attention and heightened awareness. Armed with these, a Daoist could hope to apply Wu-Wei in achieving almost any goal. *Far from being completely passive, a person using the principles of Wu-Wei is active in just the right measure at just the right time.* This is why a Tai Chi fighter can defeat an opponent with the smallest movement: nothing is ever forced or striven for. This principle of non-striving is also an unspoken 'rule' in the way we practise QSH.

There is even what we might call a 'biological' basis for the manifestation of Wu-Wei in human beings. Twentieth-century scholar-philosopher Alan Watts saw this aspect of Wu-Wei as a bio-energetic 'intelligence' embedded in our physical being: 'It [Wu-Wei] is also the "unconscious" intelligence of the whole organism and, in particular, the wisdom of the nervous system. Wu-Wei is a combination of this wisdom with taking the line of least resistance in all one's actions' (Watts 1992, p.76). Using the '"unconscious" intelligence of the whole organism' is a fine description of QSH.

Any manual techniques that are brought to bear are done so spontaneously and even then merely as a physical response to intuitions suggested by information from the patient's energy field. Such techniques are principally designed to (a) enable you, the healer, to perceive better, and (b) to, as it were, 'suggest' to the patient's Qi that it might wish to adopt a healthier configuration. This is more than enough to set the required change in motion.

Zu Ran

The Chinese term Zu Ran covers yet another highly useful Daoist insight that has become in turn a cornerstone of QSH. Zu Ran translates as something like 'by its own virtue', 'according to its intrinsic nature' or even 'all by itself'. At its most profound level, this refers to the generative principle of the universe, the spontaneous existential arising of all phenomena without any implication of a god or creator. Everything, then, ineluctably follows its own natural path, its own unique Dao.

In QSH, it is a given that Qi behaves according to Zu Ran, unless something is preventing it from doing so. We lay on hands simply to allow Qi to find its own level, to take its natural direction where something has blocked it. Yet, in sharp contrast to most other systems, we never 'tell' Qi what to do. *A QSH healer does not manipulate Qi, but merely bears witness to it and encourages it to find its own way, according to its nature.*

What you see is what you get: uses of visualization

Let us now explore another aspect of QSH, that of 'visualization'. Appropriate visualization can help the healer become aware of disruptions in the patient's Qi and gently 'encourage' a shift towards a greater level of integration. Done correctly, this is simply yet another manifestation of Wu-Wei in action. This time, however, the initial 'action' takes place within your own head. Fascinatingly, a perceptible shift in the patient's Qi field almost invariably follows. Nothing is done, and yet nothing is left undone...

Visualization for healing has always been a part of just about every ancient wisdom tradition. We are, of course, mostly interested in how Daoists have approached the subject.

Daoist visualization is an immense field, touching on martial arts, spiritual enquiry and almost every other sphere of human activity. Here we are principally concerned with what are known as 'medical meditations', visualization techniques for improving health.[1]

Unsurprisingly, Daoist medical meditation is concerned primarily with working directly with Qi. In most instances, colourful Chinese imagery – featuring tigers, dragons and the like – is used to 'trick' Qi into behaving in certain predictable ways. What this really means is that the guided imagery assists Qi in moving through particular meridian pathways or in collecting at certain energy centres. This is yet another example of the aphorism we explored in an earlier chapter, Yi Dao, Qi Dao, or 'where the mind goes, Qi follows'. Visualization, when applied like this, is definitely not just something that happens in your imagination; *it also requires you to be acutely aware of your body and your Qi.* The purpose is not to simply be in a 'good space' within your head, but rather to effect real change within your energy system (or someone else's).

QSH visualization has exactly the same goal. The major difference between QSH and mainstream Daoist medical meditation is that QSH does not employ such complex imagery, and, predictably, is much more 'passive' in its approach: Wu-Wei! Based on whatever we are perceiving about the patient's Qi, we may choose to employ visualization to make gentle 'suggestions' or otherwise encourage the energy to move or rebalance itself. We are far less concerned with opening up specific pathways or 'telling' the Qi where to go and what to do.

Remember: you might well be a highly trained therapist and a mighty healer, but actually the Qi always knows best! (A QSH visualization exercise follows at the end of this chapter.)

The mind: searchlight or daylight?

The notion of 'visualization' brings us spiralling right back to how we as QSH healers might interpret the words 'focus' and 'intent'. Once again, this is where QSH diverges from the usual Qi Gong approach. If we use our minds as a kind of ultra-focused 'searchlight', probing intensely through the patient's energy field, we will get one kind of a result. This is very much the modern EQH approach, and is arguably highly necessary for the ability to project a 'beam' of Qi into a person. However, it can also feel intrusive and tends to produce a 'tunnel vision' mentality where the practitioner's will is the most important factor. The 'bigger picture' can be missed, not to mention more subtle energetic interactions between therapist and patient. If great care is not taken, the therapist can even start to become drained; after all, they are giving away some of their Qi! However, there are other ways of focusing the mind, and the 'searchlight' mentality is only one way to be present. In QSH, our approach is very different.

If we can use the mind like a probe, we can also use it in a much more diffuse manner without losing any of its ability to effect change. To me, this is far closer to the Daoist spirit of Wu-Wei. To explain this idea, consider a different analogy. Perhaps we could view the QSH approach to achieving presence (including mental focus and visualization) as being less like a flashlight beam and more akin to the dawning of the day. Think about the similarities: the day gradually dawns, becoming ever lighter until everything is in clear view, and yet no specific object has been selected to be highlighted. The sunlight, growing in strength, illuminates everything equally, with no striving and no effort. When we sit or stand quietly by a patient's side to apply QSH, again, everything within their Qi field is gradually illuminated by our mind, with the absolute minimum of unnecessary effort. Eventually, we may be drawn to a particular area of the body or energy field where disharmony begins to announce itself to our senses, and we may begin to work on it. Even so, this has happened as the result of a quality of mind that can be likened to a kind of diffuse 'peripheral vision'.

There is nothing woolly about this. It most definitely requires us to be fully present and alert, and yet our minds are receptive, not assertive.

Let's try to get a better feel for this. The following is a QSH visualization exercise and again, requires two people, as well as a massage couch or something equivalent.

Exercise 6.1: Bringing visualization into your practice

Have the 'patient' (your partner) lie down comfortably on their back on the couch.

Sit on an upright chair close behind the patient's head.

Focus on your breathing.

Now, place both your hands, palms facing each other, about six inches either side of the patient's head. Your hands should be open and fingers separated until you feel a slight stretch in your palms.

Despite this, as in everything else in Daoism, there always remains a slight 'roundedness', a gentle curve in your fingers and at the wrists (see Figure 6.1).

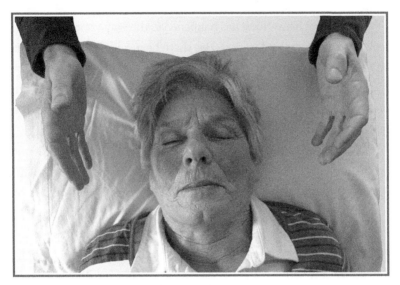

Figure 6.1: Qi Sensitivity Healing practice

You are going to be sitting almost immobile like this for a while, so it might be an idea to rest your elbows on the edge of the couch whilst you are holding your arms in this rounded posture.

Concentrate now on what you are experiencing about the patient via the medium of your hands. What does their Qi feel like? (It's fine to move your hands very slowly an inch or so in any direction that seems right to you, if that helps you perceive better. Very often it does, and you suddenly find that 'optimum spot'.)

As usual, don't analyse or judge what you are learning about your patient in this way; just do it with as little internal commentary as you can manage.

Now we are going to visualize. (We are assuming here that you know the approximate positions of the Central and Left and Right Meridians, as well as the location of the three Dan Tien.)

In your mind's eye, try to hold the image of these three meridians and Dan Tien as if they were shining with inner light (or healing mist, or whatever image works best for you). Don't try to make the energy do anything! Just continue to picture it. If your mind wanders and you lose focus, it's not a disaster; just gently return to your visualization. Keep this up for at least five minutes.

Now notice if anything has happened to the way your patient's Qi feels in your palms and fingers. Has there been a shift of any kind? Is anything different now?

Has the patient changed in any other way, such as how they are breathing? Have they let out any deep sighs, or 'sunk' further into the fabric of the couch in relaxation?

Do you have any sudden intuitions or insights about the patient or their health? Have you acquired any information about them that might affect the way you treat them with, say, Acupuncture or massage?

And what has happened to you yourself during this process? Do you feel in any way different? Has your relationship with the patient undergone any subtle shift? Do you feel more compassionate towards them, or do you perhaps feel like you understand them better as a person? Do you feel energetically 'connected'?

These are just suggestions of what can happen when you are visualizing. Perhaps sometimes nothing much seems to happen. As usual I advise you first to relax and then just to practise, practise, practise! Remember also that absolutely everybody has the potential to develop healing hands. If that is a natural human birthright, why would you be any different?

The following chapters will lay out for you what I regard as the core techniques of QSH, including some more applications for visualization.

Notes

1.   The American Qi Gong master Kenneth Cohen has been particularly influential in bringing this type of medical meditation to the notice of Westerners.

Chapter 7

QSH TECHNIQUES PART 1: TURNING THEORY INTO THERAPY

So far we have looked very closely at the mindset or 'philosophy' of QSH as a healing modality, as well as how it is intended to dovetail with the most fundamental ideas of traditional Daoism. By now we should have also acquired some feel for how it differs from other, more familiar therapies. The exercises encountered so far have been designed principally as preparation, a solid foundation on which we can begin to build refined healing skills over an entire lifetime.

We have also looked in some detail already at how QSH is not really a technique-based discipline, but rather a method of bringing about positive energetic shifts in another human being by means of a heightened sense of awareness – which is really just another way of saying that we must cultivate the ability to maintain relaxed presence at all times. (This apparent passivity brings to mind that old Buddhist meditation joke, 'Don't just do something: sit there!') To a great extent, just sitting or standing in a state of heightened awareness really is how we practise QSH, but even so this is by no means the entire story.

We have already encountered a few examples of how the judicious use of hand positions, breathing techniques and visualization can enhance the clinical effectiveness of QSH. I don't normally like to think of these as 'techniques' as such; most of them are better described as spontaneous responses to kinetically perceived imbalances in the patient's energy. At no point during a treatment do I ever say to myself: 'Ah, now I am going to use techniques A, B and Z whilst simultaneously employing Visualization No. 3.' Instead, these things are allowed simply to happen of their own accord, and I have never in the past felt the need to assign names or labels to them.

Despite this in-the-moment, unplanned quality that is built into QSH, in this chapter and the next I will attempt to catalogue the most common of the 'manoeuvres' and visualizations that I find myself making in the clinic, so that they can be assimilated and learned in a systematic way. Whilst this goes a little against the grain, it is done here purely for the sake of convenience in passing the information on to you, the reader. Therefore, for the moment we shall just go ahead and use the term 'techniques'. What follows is in no way a definitive list of the techniques that I have created for use in my own clinical practice, and you must also feel free to adapt what you learn here, should you feel the need. You might even go so far as to create some techniques of your own. I'd be fascinated to see what you come up with!

Before we start to learn any specific protocols, however, now is probably the right time to review the core values of QSH. It should go without saying that everything you learn in this chapter and the next is to be considered within the context of these values.

We can say that any QSH treatment contains all of the following:

- an understanding of correct posture and structural alignment

- mindful breathing

- visualization

- the spontaneous application of hands, on or off the body

- the ability to summon and maintain continuous presence

- an intuitive, kinetically based understanding of a patient's Qi

- a non-invasive, non-manipulative approach at all times

- a relaxed, 'passive' and receptive mindset.

We can also state that whilst it takes discipline and practice to perform, QSH's bias is nonetheless emphatically towards the non-intellectual and non-analytical. It is not based on any formal system of diagnosis. Instead, it models itself on the Daoist principles of naturalness and Wu-Wei.

Finally, we note once more the unusual feature that QSH can always be performed as just one component of any existing treatment regime, at one and the same time as that other treatment.

You can perform QSH whilst Acupuncture needles are in situ, or whilst giving Shiatsu, Swedish massage, osteopathy or indeed almost any other kind of bodywork. QSH simply moulds itself around whatever diagnosis and treatment strategy a practitioner has been trained to produce, with no contradiction. In other circumstances it can also be used as a stand-alone system in its own right.

Before we begin to learn any specific techniques, however, I'd like to talk a little more about the meaning of De Qi, and its prime relevance to our practice as healers.

De Qi: what it is and how to achieve it

The Chinese words De Qi can be translated loosely as 'the ability to make contact with the Qi of another person in such a way as to bring about a desired change in their energy'. In fact, the manifestation of De Qi is regarded as essential in many aspects of Chinese Medicine, especially Acupuncture. QSH is no different in this respect, and in

Part 1 of Exercise 7.1 we are going to learn how to achieve De Qi consistently with the earth itself. This is an essential skill, not only in QSH but also in such traditional disciplines as Qi Gong and, most particularly, Nei Gong.

Some more theory might be useful here. Anyone interested in Daoism will know that the Chinese word for a human being, Ran, translates as 'between Heaven and Earth'. This was meant to be understood in two ways. First, a human was seen as the amalgamation of spiritual energies filtering down from the cosmos with a more earthy physicality that was very much the product of this particular planet. This amalgamation allowed humans, uniquely, to become (at least potentially) wise, thinking creatures capable of spiritual evolution. At the same time, such beings were still firmly embedded in the reality of physical existence and fully capable of action in that sphere.

The second meaning of Ran is purely about Qi. Yang heavenly Qi (Tian Qi) and Yin earthly Qi (Di Qi) were seen as complementary opposites that, once again, blended with each other to form not only human life but also everything else that we see around us. Heavenly Qi had no religious meaning as such, but referred instead to the refined Yang Qi of deep space, plus the Qi-laden oxygen of the sky. Earthly Qi, on the other hand, was the denser, more Yin Qi, emanating primarily from the earth's magnetic core. To be human was to be the crucible in which occurred a dynamic interchange of both of these types of Qi, and a great many protocols in Qi Gong and Nei Gong were carefully designed to amplify this natural process.

So, when we talk about 'grounding' in those disciplines and in QSH, we really mean making a conscious link with the great, swirling reservoir of Qi held deep inside the earth. This idea is intended to be taken literally, not metaphorically.

Why do we need to do this? There are several very good reasons. First, earthly Qi penetrates our body principally through the feet, and in particular through the acupoint Yong Quan (KD 1), also known as 'Bubbling Stream'. This powerful vertical flow of Qi is energizing to the entire human system, so clearly the better the upward flow, the more robust and healthy will we become.

The second reason for achieving a strong, continuous De Qi connection with the Earth is that it enables the healer to act as a kind of 'lightning rod' or electrical earth wire to keep both themselves and the patient clear of toxic Qi (Xie Qi). In reality, toxic Qi tends to sink slowly downwards like a heavy gas rather than shooting like a lightning bolt. Either way, this is why we always keep our feet on the ground, both metaphorically and literally!

Now for some technical learning. The following exercises are designed as partner work, and require a treatment couch or similar. Unless stated otherwise, they can all be performed either sitting or standing.

Exercise 7.1, Part 1: De Qi for grounding

Assume a comfortable QSH posture, close to your patient.

Tune in to your breathing.

Now take your mind down into the soles of your feet, which should be in firm contact with the floor. Take at least a minute or two to experience whatever you find there. (It is quite likely at this stage that acupoint Yong Quan (KD 1) will begin to announce its presence. This might be felt as a strong tingling, or even as something indefinable spiralling up through the legs. This is all to the good, but don't worry if not much appears to be happening at Yong Quan, because the grounding process will still be working. Sometimes the sensations are much more diffuse and experienced throughout the feet or legs.)

Now visualize roots, or tendrils, emanating from Yong Quan and beginning to penetrate into the ground. Without any strain or undue effort, use your mind to gently drive these roots ever deeper into the earth. At the same time the roots should start to spread out, as if supporting a mighty tree. The watchwords here are deep and wide.

(A note about projecting your mind into the earth: it is never enough just to say to oneself, for instance, 'Australia!' and have your Qi immediately arrive there. Nor can you just picture the moon or stars and have your Qi go there instantaneously. The mind has to calmly lead the Qi all the way. So when we are grounding ourselves and seeking De Qi with the earth's core, we really do need to visualize our 'roots' penetrating through floorboards, the foundations of whatever building we are in, and through soil, clay and rock. A good visual imagination helps, not to mention the ability to maintain a relaxed focus. Lead the Qi down as deep and as widely as you can, but do not strain! In reality, if you extend down beyond your own energy field (about a metre in most people), you will be contacting the earthly Qi anyway.)

Now notice how visualizing in this way has changed the quality of your contact with the floor. Do your feet and lower body feel somehow different? Heavier perhaps? Tingly? More alive?

We can enhance this contact if we so desire. This is only really applicable if we are using just one hand to heal with (something I tend to do quite often), and therefore have one hand free.

With your free hand, adopt the hand posture detailed in Figure 7.1. The second or third finger is dropped, so that it points to the floor. (It doesn't appear to matter which of these fingers you use, although I myself seem to favour the third.) Bring your mind to the finger, and imagine Qi sinking and spiralling softly downwards from its tip. Note whatever you experience.

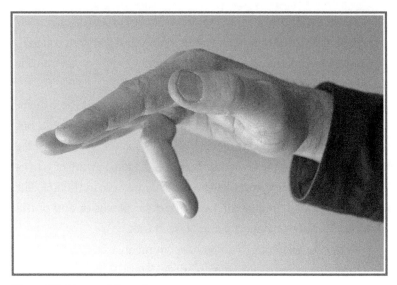

Figure 7.1: 'Dropped finger'

Now imagine the earthly Qi rising lazily up to meet the Qi from your finger. Remember that Qi tends to obey the bidding of your mind, as long as you are focused. Can you feel the moment that contact is made, almost as if something has just 'turned itself on'?

Whenever it seems appropriate (with practice you will know this intuitively), use this hand shape both to enhance your De Qi with the ground and to act as the 'lightning rod' that offloads Xie Qi. Although you may find very similar techniques to this in Qi Gong, it is again context that is the most important element here. In this case, we are not achieving De Qi as a prelude to a conscious, pre-planned manipulation of the other person's Qi.

Now, in Part 2 of the exercise, we are going to practise gaining De Qi with the patient's energy field.

Exercise 7.1, Part 2: Establishing De Qi with your patient

Have your 'patient' lie down, face upwards, on the treatment couch.

Stand and breathe in the required manner until your mind is settled and receptive.

Using one hand to sense with, move slowly around the patient, feeling for imbalances in their energy field. (Remember: you do not need to know what these imbalances mean, or have any concrete idea of what you are going to do about them. Just become aware of what's there, that's all. Such distortions can occur anywhere in the EEF, but around the general area of the head, the solar plexus or any of the three Dan Tien are extremely common scenarios.)

Let's say, for example, that you have found an area over the solar plexus, roughly in the region of acupoint Jiu Wei (CV 15), that seems to you slightly cold, and somehow empty, a place where the Qi does not feel vital. Somehow you are 'attracted' to work on this area. In fact, it might even feel that, once your mind became calm enough, your hand was just led there, as if it just 'knew' where to go.

Now sit or stand close by the side of your client.

Assume the 'Dropped Finger' hand posture detailed in Exercise 7.1, Part 1. Become aware of the connection between your hand and the Qi of the earth. (Visualize this too, if it helps, but remember that it is far more important to actually *feel* than it is to imagine.) Feel the connection through your feet too.

Once you are feeling a high-quality De Qi connection with both the patient and the earth, ask the patient if would be alright for you to gently place the palm of one hand on the their body, at the place where you noticed their imbalance (see Figure 7.2). Accuracy is not paramount here, as you are using your entire palm.

Just leave your hand on the patient's body, as you 'meditate' on their Qi. Soon you may become aware of many sensations that you had not noticed at first: pulsing, tingling, warmth, a sense of 'movement', perhaps, that is purely energetic. It may feel as if something powerful just 'switched on' within the patient. This moment, once experienced, is unmistakeable, and usually precedes an increasingly insistent, rhythmic 'pulsing' that has nothing to do with the pulsing of the blood. Be careful NOT to analyse this process and do NOT consciously attempt to change whatever you are perceiving in any way. Being aware is enough.

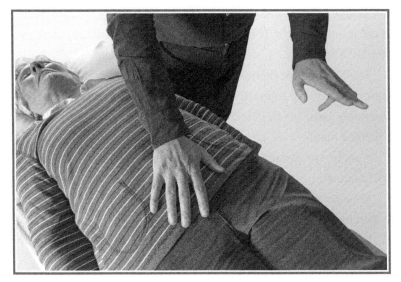

Figure 7.2: Achieving De Qi

After a minute or two (or five!), you will tend to realize that the task is somehow done. The area you have been focused on now feels mysteriously more functional and coherent. The Qi has changed, although you may not be able to put into words exactly what has altered. You don't have to! You may also notice that there has been a change in the patient too. Perhaps they are calmer, breathing more deeply, a better colour, or simply more relaxed.

Now, in the same way as above, move on to any other part of the EEF that feels 'wrong' to you and repeat the process. Do this until the entire EEF appears to be more integrated and whole.

At this point you could resume your Acupuncture, Shiatsu or whatever therapy you were practising at the same time as the QSH healing.

Exercise 7.2: 'Smoothing out' the external energy field

This exercise admittedly is one of just a few that come as close to being 'interventions' as QSH ever can. Nevertheless, context and intent are everything: we tend to apply this technique spontaneously, without any premeditation, and simply because it is what our hands 'want to do'. In other words, it is intuition-based and, at best, bypasses the intellect altogether.

This is why I see this manoeuvre, and a few others that are in the same category, not so much as interventions but as means by which we simply assist the Qi in reconfiguring itself naturally – literally just a 'helping hand'.

Assume the familiar standing posture and breathe in the usual QSH manner.

Now move around the patient, sensing with your hands as you did in Exercise 7.1, Part 2.

Let your hands guide you to where the EEF seems in some way dysfunctional.

Using the now-familiar hand posture and awareness of your contact with the ground through your feet, allow yourself to feel a sense of De Qi with the earth.

With the other hand (the 'healing hand') palm open, achieve De Qi with your patient's EEF.

Now, in the most relaxed way possible and without using your mind as a searchlight, allow the healing hand to start making small circles around the area you have been drawn to. This motion is very much like cleaning a dirty window with a cloth, so long as it is slow and gentle and never vigorous.

Keep performing this easy, almost lazy motion until you feel a definite change for the better in the patient's EEF. You will know when this has happened, as it will feel as if you have 'smoothed out' an area that was anything but smooth before you started.

Continue until that part of the EEF feels 'healed', and then either move on to another area or return to the therapy you were practising alongside QSH.

A few thoughts about hand direction...

In some healing modalities, and Qi Gong's EQH is definitely one of them, great attention is paid to the direction in which one rotates one's hands or fingers during healing. In EQH, this is said to greatly affect the outcome, by manipulating the Qi in very specific ways. This is parallel to TCM-style needling techniques in Acupuncture, where a clockwise rotation of the needle is thought to tonify (strengthen) Qi, whilst counter-clockwise is said to reduce excessive Qi. It is not so in QSH, because, as we know, we are not trying to manipulate Qi in such a conscious manner in the first place. It is also my personal experience that whilst this might work in Acupuncture, it does not seem to make a great deal of difference in hands-on/off healing, unless you have a specific agenda for the Qi in the first place. My advice is to use your hand motions merely to smooth or encourage Qi to find its own way to wholeness. If you approach healing with this mindset, the precise direction of your movements will not greatly matter.

In Chapter 8 that follows we will explore some more in-depth QSH techniques.

Chapter 8

QSH TECHNIQUES PART 2: GOING INSIDE

In this chapter I want to detail some slightly more sophisticated, or, at the very least, slightly more demanding, QSH techniques that I use regularly in the clinic. They are sophisticated not because they are complex, but in the sense that they often require an even more heightened ability to perceive Qi than in the exercises we have encountered so far. Mastering these techniques will not only take you deeper into your practical understanding of QSH, but will also quite literally allow you to fully penetrate the vast network of energetic circuitry that lies within the core of the human body. They are valuable clinical tools.

Healing hands or healing hand?

At this point we should be thinking in terms of exactly what we are doing with each hand.

Although many QSH techniques call for both hands to be working on a patient simultaneously, most do not. This is important because I have noticed that the majority of us lead either with the right or the left hand when we are giving healing. A few individuals are 'ambidextrous' in this respect. We seem to know instinctively which hand is best suited for healing, and which to use in a supportive function. Interestingly, the hand of choice is not always the one we use in everyday activities. I have seen right-handed people favour their left hand in healing, and vice versa. Just experiment to find what works best for you.

Engaging with the meridian system

As we have already seen in our investigation of traditional meridian theory, the Qi flows within the human body can be categorized as follows:

- 12 medical acquired meridians

- eight congenital/extraordinary meridians (also called the 'eight extraordinary vessels')

- the 'trinity' of the Central, Left and Right Meridians. (You may remember from an earlier chapter that this separate category has been created purely for functional purposes.)

We are now going to learn how to access the 12 medical acquired meridians of a patient, using QSH methodology.

Exercise 8.1: 'Opening' a meridian

At this stage you should be well acquainted with what is required in terms of breathing, posture and attaining De Qi, both with the ground and with the patient. For the sake of brevity, from this point on we shall just assume that each of these preliminaries has been done at the start of each exercise. All the exercises in this chapter require a partner and a treatment couch.

In QSH, the best way to open any specified meridian is via one or more of its acupoints.

The following three protocols are really just variants on this theme. They can be applied to any of the medical acquired meridians or the Du and Ren Mai, but in order to learn them, it is probably best to confine ourselves to just one hypothetical problem. In this example I have selected the Stomach Meridian to demonstrate typical QSH approaches to meridian and acupoint issues.

So, let us say that you are in session with a patient, and that you have been running your 'sensing' hand about four inches or so above their body, searching for disharmony.

Somewhere about halfway down one of the shins, let's imagine you start to perceive a disturbance in the Qi, an imbalance of some kind.

As usual, you do not need to analyse this imbalance or give it a name, but you do need to deal with it. Bringing your palm (or perhaps even one or more of your fingers) closer to the patient's leg, you determine that the dysfunction seems to lie somewhere within the Stomach Meridian, at approximately the site of acupoint Feng Long (ST 40).

You do not need to consider the functions of the Stomach Meridian, or of the acupoint in question. Just for now, set all such theoretical knowledge aside if you can. However, as your intuition is nevertheless telling you to engage with this acupoint, you now have a range of options...

Technique A: 'Hovering palm'

You could allow your palm to 'hover' over the acupoint, making small, gentle circles, as you learned in Chapter 7. At the same time, with the other hand you are seeking to maintain conscious De Qi with the ground using either the 'Open Palm' or 'Dropped Finger' technique you learned in Chapter 7. Meditate on what you are experiencing via the medium of your hands.

You now have the additional option to visualize healthy Qi as it might manifest at the acupoint, or, better still, as it might move smoothly through the entire length of the meridian. I find it appropriate to visualize this Qi in the colours described in the 'Theory of the Five Elements'.[1] As we are dealing with the Stomach Meridian here, the Qi would be a healthy Earth element yellow.

Continue sensing and visualizing in this way until you feel that characteristic yet inexplicable change occur as the patient's energy awakens, first at the acupoint in question and then possibly also as a ripple effect down the meridian or even throughout the energetic system as a whole. You will most certainly recognize this when it happens.

Technique B: 'Pulling threads'

Follow the instructions in Technique A above, only this time don't use the 'Hovering palm' method. Instead, form the fingers of your healing hand into a loose 'beak' (see Figure 8.1).

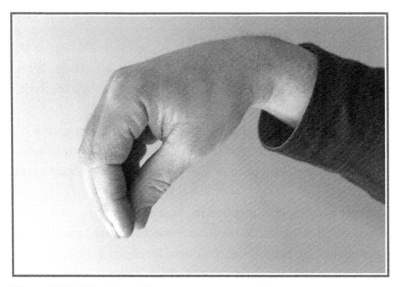

Figure 8.1: 'Pulling threads'

With the fingers of this beak, start to make slow, gentle spirals above the acupoint, about one to four inches off the patient's skin. You should soon begin to feel a connection between your fingers and the acupoint. The Qi here will probably feel dysfunctional in some way or other.

(Language is not particularly helpful to us here. These sensations are extremely subjective, but nevertheless very real.)

'Take hold' of this dysfunctional Qi as if it were a bunch of invisible threads. Mindfully, begin to pull these threads out of the patient. This can take a minute or two, and it is quite common for both of you to feel this happening. Once you are sure that the energetic imbalance has been removed at the acupoint, return to the 'Hovering palm' technique to smooth out this portion of the EEF.

Alternatively, you could employ either of two slightly more powerful, hands-on variants of the above. These are my main techniques for dealing with acupoints, or for any very small, localized areas of Qi imbalance. (The hands-off, open-palm technique is best suited for dealing with wider, more general areas of imbalance, or for disturbances within the EEF.)

Technique C: 'Sensing finger'

Select one hand to be your 'healing' hand. Use whichever finger from this hand feels most right to you to find and lightly touch the dysfunctional acupoint.[2]

Maintain this light contact of finger and acupoint (see Figure 8.2).

At the same time, use the other hand to gain De Qi with the ground. Again, either the 'Open palm' or the 'Dropped finger' technique will work here.

Now, standing or sitting in a meditative state, bring your mind to bear on the acupoint. Do this in as gentle and relaxed a manner as you possibly can, but preferably without letting your mind drift off. Remember, in QSH the mind is clear and firm, but it is not to be used like a searchlight, even when it is meditating on a relatively localized physical area.

If you wish, visualize the appropriate colour of the meridian.

Eventually, you will feel how the acupoint 'opens up' to your finger. This opening is something that happens quite suddenly and spontaneously, and occurs on two distinct levels.

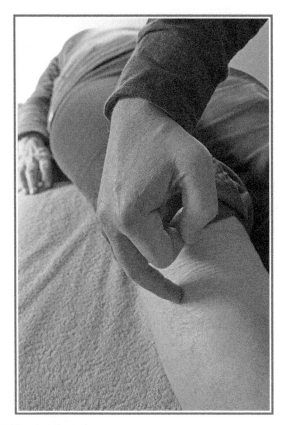

Figure 8.2: 'Sensing finger'

On the physical level, the acupoint will tend to feel 'tight' at first, but eventually it will unfurl, rather like the petals of a flower. You will suddenly find that your finger is penetrating deeper into the surrounding tissue, and that the characteristic saucer-shaped 'mouth' of the acupoint has become significantly wider. There will be a palpable relaxation of the local musculature.

Please ensure that you are not achieving this by simply pressing harder. Any physical contact with the acupoint should always be absolutely minimal: we are not performing acupressure here!

The second, most important, level of this opening-up tends to occur spontaneously and in tandem with the physical relaxation around the acupoint. This is a purely energetic phenomenon. The acupoint will 'wake up' and begin to pulsate in a very obvious way.

Be sure that you really are feeling the energy change and not just the pulsing of the blood in your own finger! In reality, the two sensations are quite different, and with practice you will never be likely to get them mixed up.

Healthy Qi feels very different from sick or blocked Qi. These feelings are subtle and subjective, but absolutely real. We could use descriptors such as 'fresh', 'flowing' or 'clean', as opposed to 'stagnant', 'sticky' or 'random', but, of course, these are just words. You will instinctively know when a higher-quality emanation of Qi makes its presence felt, and at such times words become redundant.

Experience this more coherent energy flow for a minute or two, and then move on to something else.

Technique D: 'Distal grip'

This is exactly the same as Technique B, but with one important difference.

This time, you will use the 'healing' hand in exactly the same way as described above, but with the other hand you will not be seeking De Qi with the ground. Instead, use the soles of your feet for this.

Now ask the patient's permission to use your free hand to lightly grasp their body at a location further down the meridian you are working on. In the case of the Stomach Meridian, this would be the second toe. However, in QSH you really don't need to be that specific. Just take a firm but gentle hold of the patient's foot, or even the ankle, wrapping your entire hand around it if you can (see Figure 8.3). You will now be covering several acupoints at once.

Now patiently wait for the energy to activate, as described above. Remember, by freeing up acupoints in this way, you are going a long way towards freeing up their related meridians too. This in turn will tend to produce a positive knock-on effect throughout the energy body.

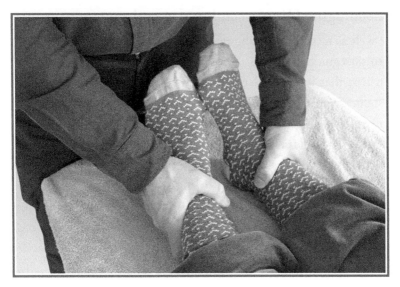

Figure 8.3: 'Distal grip'

In my opinion, Technique D is the most potent of these three variants for opening up acupoints and meridians. I originally developed it as a means of mimicking the TCM Acupuncture protocol of selecting a 'distal point' to support treatment that was going on further along a meridian. These distal points therefore tend to be located at the body's extremities, especially at the hands and feet. The idea here is that in using a distal point (or, in QSH, simply a distal handhold) we can excite and motivate the Qi within a meridian to move in a more powerful manner than could be achieved by merely treating the area local to the perceived problem. To do this, you need to know the direction of travel that Qi takes within the meridian in question.[3] In our example here, the Stomach Qi normally travels downwards from the head towards the toes, so, in general, a distal point for the Stomach should be selected from the area of the feet. In a sense, this is rather like dredging a blocked watercourse. Qi does indeed often behave in a very similar way to liquid – hence all the water imagery in Daoist energy arts.

Encouraging Qi to ascend or descend

As well as targeting specific meridians or acupoints whenever our intuition guides us to, we can influence Qi in a much more general sense so that it flows relatively unhindered throughout the entire system. This can be very powerful. I have come to realize that the potency of such techniques almost certainly lies in their ability to activate significant elements of the congenital meridians and even the 'trinity' meridians.

Again, working at this level is not something that we plan. It simply happens when the Qi 'tells' us it should. In scanning over a patient's energetic anatomy with our hands, we may have a sudden insight that Qi is generally just not flowing either upwards or downwards in the way it should. We don't need to know why. Sometimes, of course, signs and symptoms also suggest that this might be occurring, even before we have undertaken a scan. A flushed face and migraine headache often tells us that Yang Qi is not fully able to descend from the head, for example. In QSH, we allow such things to help us form a good general impression of how the patient's energy is behaving, but beyond that we don't worry about the specifics.

In humans and many other creatures, energy describes an 'oval' – up the back and down the front of the body, following the pathways of the 'Governing Vessel' (Du Mai) and 'Conception Vessel' (Ren Mai). In Daoism this well-known pathway is, of course, called the 'Microcosmic Orbit', or sometimes the 'Small Heavenly Circulation'. It is principally this that we will be working with here. Another way of looking at this orbit is to remember that at its most basic level it is really just an interchange of Yang (rising) and Yin (descending) energies.

Exercise 8.2: 'Knife hand' body sweep

I have named this protocol after a common Oriental martial arts technique, the 'Knife hand', which is also sometimes colloquially known as a 'karate chop' here in the West. The resemblance is entirely superficial! (See Figure 8.4.)

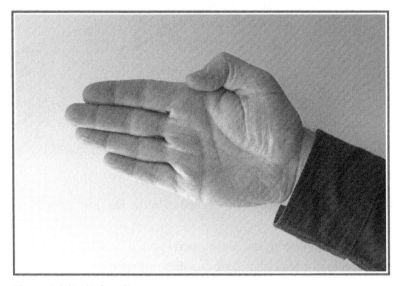

Figure 8.4: 'Knife hand'

With your 'patient' lying on their back on the couch, stand by their side, roughly on a level with their head and neck.

Gain De Qi with one hand, and with the other hand assume the 'Knife hand' posture.

Now, keeping your 'Knife hand' roughly four inches above the patient, begin slowly and mindfully to 'sweep' down the entire length of the body, approximately over the pathway of Ren Mai ('Conception Vessel') (see Figure 8.5).

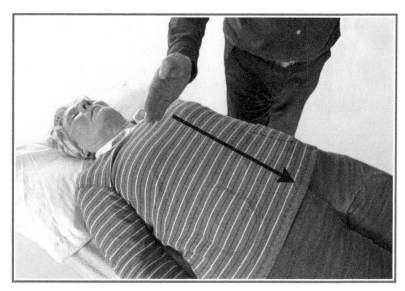

Figure 8.5: 'Knife hand body sweep'

If, or rather *when*, you feel a dysfunction in the EEF, just allow your hand to stop moving.

This is admittedly an odd phenomenon; it is almost as if the hand comes to a dead stop above any place where there is significant imbalance. (This is often within deeper energetic structures, rather than acupoints or surface meridians.) No decision to make the hand stop like this has been made; it happens all by itself. This is not easy to master, as it really does require the mind to be very still, reflecting what it perceives like a mirror.

Once your hand has hit this invisible 'obstruction' in the EEF, employ a combination of the 'Hovering palm' and 'Smoothing out' techniques you have already learned to encourage it to dissipate.

Now continue with 'Knife hand' further down the body until you hit the next obstruction.

Clear the obstruction and move on down. Continue to do this until you feel you can sweep slowly down from the patient's head to their toes without encountering anything that feels energetically 'wrong' to you.

The entire EEF down the front of the body should now feel uniformly healthy and free-flowing. It's also quite possible that the patient will have begun to register changes too, perhaps even an improvement in symptoms.

Now ask the patient to turn over so that they are lying face down. Repeat the entire 'knife hand/sweeping' process along their body, although this time you are sweeping *upwards*, from the feet to the head, and paying particular attention to Qi obstructions in the spinal column.

(You will probably also need to employ the 'Sensing finger' technique on imbalanced acupoints along the Bladder and Du Meridians, as well as on Hua Tuo Jia Ji points on either side of the spine.)

Exercise 8.4: Streaming the Qi downwards

This is a potent but relatively easy technique that greatly facilitates the downward flow of Qi.

I use it frequently, either with patients who tell me they are too much 'in their head', as in, for example, cases of anxiety, or simply to ground Qi safely at the end of a treatment. This tends to have a profoundly calming effect on the patient, and also helps to keep the therapist's own Qi field clear of energetic pollution.

Stand or sit at the foot of the treatment couch and take hold of the patient's feet. The precise handhold isn't important, although I tend to favour placing a thumb lightly on each Yong Quan (KD 1) acupoint at the same time placing one or more fingers around the area of acupoint Tai Chong (LV 3). There is no need to press (see Figure 8.6).

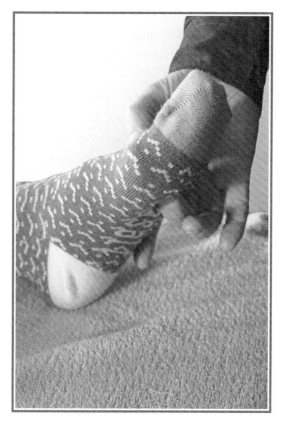

Figure 8.6: 'Streaming the Qi downwards'

Spend a minute or two meditating on the patient's Qi.

When the Qi begins to feel more stable, finish the technique off with the following visualization. This can make a *huge* difference!

Visualize the entire room that you are working in as a sea of energy, coming up to about the level of where the patient is lying on the treatment couch. If it helps, give this 'sea' a colour, gentle waves, or whatever will make it easier to keep it in focus. I tend to picture it as warm water. Your hands remain in contact with the patient's feet throughout.

Now, slowly but surely, watch with your mind's eye as the level of this 'sea' slowly subsides, draining effortlessly downwards into the floor. You may feel Qi descending through your legs and feet. Make sure it continues to sink deep into the earth, until the process feels completed.

(This ensures it has gone safely beyond the bounds of your personal energy field.)

Exercise 8.5: Visualizing the descending flow

Another of my favourites, this technique is again easy to perform but potentially extremely useful in both helping Qi to descend the length of the patient's body and in calming a busy or distressed mind.

It is an especially useful technique for acupuncturists in particular, as it can be done whilst the patient is lying on the treatment couch with needles retained.

Sit or stand behind the patient's head and place your hands underneath them, palms open, at the approximate bilateral locations of either Tian Zhu (UB 10) on the neck, or Feng Men (UB 12) on the upper back. I often spend several minutes holding each area.

Feel the characteristic bilateral 'pulsing' as the acupoints throughout the entire area become active.

Now visualize the Central, Left and Right Meridians (the 'trinity') and the three Dan Tien, glowing with energy.

With your mind, gently 'ask' the patient's Qi to descend. Watch it as it passes down the meridians and through these three major energy entres.

Once the Qi has flowed out beyond the feet (beyond a metre is about right), the technique is completed.

Exercise 8.6: Symptomatic healing

It will often be the case that someone who is otherwise reasonably balanced and healthy presents with a purely symptomatic, muscular-skeletal issue. This could be anything from an arthritic knee or frozen shoulder to a twisted ankle, and would normally fall under the Chinese Medicine category of 'localized stagnation of Blood and Qi'. By way of example, let's say we're dealing here with a case of tennis elbow. The QSH protocol is beautifully simple.

Standing or sitting beside the patient, wrap both hands gently around the affected area.

Hold, experience and meditate until there is a distinct enlivening of the Qi and Blood throughout the entire area. Wait until this flow is strong and even. Pain may intensify slightly at this point; do not panic! Reassure your patient that it is all part of the process and keep going until the discomfort subsides. This usually takes just a few minutes. (Obviously, in the exceptional case where the pain becomes really acute during healing, then stop! There is clearly something very wrong and you should refer this person to a doctor immediately.)

Assuming all is going well, check with the patient that there has been a change in symptoms, such as enhanced movement or a decrease in pain. (In practice, you might also want to bring the 'Sensing finger' technique to bear on acupoints in the affected area. I generally use both these QSH techniques on a muscular-skeletal issue, during the same treatment session in which I might also use Acupuncture, Tui Na or both.)

In the final chapter I am going to present a few case studies to give you an even better grasp of how QSH can be applied, and how it can be seamlessly merged with your existing therapeutic skills. I will also detail some highly important methods for preventing yourself from becoming ill as a result of transferring sick Qi from the patient's energy field to your own.

Notes

1. Like Yin-Yang Theory, the Theory of the Five Elements (Wu Xing) is a fundamental cornerstone of traditional Chinese thought. Originating in the Warring States period, (476–221 BCE), the theory has waxed and waned repeatedly in its popularity, and has been used over the centuries as a diagnostic tool in every walk of life, from martial arts to political prognostication and, of course, medicine.

The word 'elements' can be a source of confusion, as for Westerners the word tends to denote building blocks of matter, as in modern chemistry. It is probably far more helpful to think of Wu Xing as the 'Five Transformations', or 'Five Phases of Energy'. Looked at this way, the theory describes a predictable cycle of energetic metamorphosis, in which one aspect of Qi will predominate at any given time. The phases are named Earth, Metal, Water, Wood and Fire, each of which helps to keep the others in a state of dynamic balance via a complex set of correspondences. Disharmony is said to occur wherever this balance is interrupted. Entire systems of healing have been based upon Wu Xing, notably in the fields of Acupuncture and Shiatsu.

2. In a great many healing traditions, from Mexican Curandero healing right through to Daoist Qi Gong, healing Qi is said to be projected best from the region of the centre of the palms. Specifically, this corresponds to acupoint Lao Gong (PC 8). Perhaps it is the Pericardium Meridian's connection with the compassionate and expansive qualities of the Fire element that makes this so. Interestingly enough, in QSH I have always naturally tended to use my second finger for connecting with a patient's acupoints. This, like so much in QSH, just 'came about', and yet it does definitely seem to be both the most comfortable and most powerful finger to use in this way. Perhaps the Pericardium Meridian, terminating at that finger, provides the explanation...

3. In fact, a meridian is not quite the uni-directional entity that many people believe it to be. Information, in the form of Qi, can pass in either direction, and in ways that are not always dysfunctional. I have heard this described as being rather like a telephone wire that allows for two-way communication. Nevertheless, there is most definitely a 'preferred direction' of flow within each meridian, and in the vast majority of clinical applications it is clearly safest and best to encourage Qi to move in this way.

Chapter 9

INTEGRATION

Applying Qi Sensitivity Healing in the clinic

In this final chapter we are going to examine the 'nuts and bolts' of how QSH can be successfully integrated with one's existing therapy, be it Acupuncture, Shiatsu, Tui Na or some other modality. Practical example strikes me as the most effective way to convey this information, and so later in the chapter there will be a number of detailed case studies.

Before we approach the case studies, however, there is still one major aspect of QSH (or, indeed, any other kind of healing) that needs to be focused on at all times. This is what I would call 'energy hygiene', or, slightly less succinctly, 'how not to become ill, or make your patients ill, whilst giving healing'.

It seems to me that energy hygiene is often spoken of (even when we don't use these exact words), but nevertheless practised infrequently amongst the complementary medicine community. This is a mistake. I have witnessed energetic 'burnout' in a number of colleagues of various disciplines, some of it so severe that the practitioner had to cease treating patients for quite a time. Less severe cases seemed to involve miscellaneous symptoms such as unaccountable exhaustion or depression, headaches, anxiety, dizziness, palpitations or simply a pervasive feeling of being ungrounded or imbalanced. Of course, there might be many reasons why a therapist might become suddenly unwell, but here I am speaking only of those occasions where inadequate energy hygiene was the chief suspect. (Generally, the practitioners themselves seemed blissfully unaware of this having happened to them.) So why are complementary therapists apparently somewhat prone to this fundamental error?

Although I think there may be multiple answers to our question, it seems to me that the following issues in particular stand out:

- *Inadequate training.* I have (unfortunately) witnessed therapists draining their patients and vice versa. They were unaware this was happening and did not even consider the possibility because their training had taught them that their particular therapy was entirely benevolent and therefore safe.

- *Naivety.* Many practitioners do indeed make sincere efforts to maintain their energetic integrity on behalf of the client. However, sometimes their precautions are simply not up to the job. It is naive indeed to think that, for example, burning a sage smudge sick in the therapy room is going to prevent energetic problems from arising – at least potentially – if one is dealing with extremely ill or imbalanced individuals. Nor is opening a window, or surrounding yourself and the client in a visualized blue bubble 'for protection' going to be of very great service if, for instance, your client has something so energetically draining as, say, terminal cancer or severe mental illness. As with all aspects of healing, the rule should always be: if in doubt – don't.

- *Lack of awareness.* Training your sensitivity to Qi is absolutely vital. You need to be able to feel if, for instance, your patient's sick Qi is clinging to your hands, or, even worse, has started to creep up your forearms. You should know the precise moment when you lose De Qi with the patient, or with the floor. It's vital that you can sense the patient's Qi increasing in volume and/or balance during the treatment. If the opposite is happening, you should be in a position to know about it immediately and either adjust what you are doing or just stop. Being able to feel your own Qi flowing away unbidden into the patient is also a key skill. You should also know exactly what to do to remedy any of these situations. It all comes down to one thing: awareness.

- *Ego.* Make no mistake about it, ego is *the* main cause of problems with energy hygiene. In fact, I would say that, in every respect, overcoming one's ego is the single most significant challenge any healer has to face. Ego can manifest in many, many ways, such as the case of the healer who takes pride in experiencing their patients' illnesses in his or her own body. This isn't empathy – this is ego exploiting a basic misunderstanding about how easily dysfunctional Qi can 'infect' another person. It's certainly nothing to be proud of!

Once you start thinking that you are somehow special or, worse, that you have unusual or unique healing powers, then you might just have a problem! Anybody can give healing.

The only thing about your status as a healer that is 'special' is that you have taken the time to learn how to do it safely and well.

So what's the best way to employ energy hygiene? As usual in QSH, it's best to think less in terms of techniques and to focus more on awareness and intent. *In fact, this book has already provided you with just about everything you need to know to maintain the integrity of your Qi.* For a QSH healer, this implies:

- ongoing cultivation of a heightened sensitivity to Qi

- ability to tell the difference between your client's Qi and your own

- use of posture and breathing to establish a strong and clear flow of Qi

- awareness of precisely what is happening within the Qi fields of both patient and therapist at all times, requiring a relaxed, but constant focus

- ability to stay grounded – in other words, you must always be able to gain, and maintain, De Qi with the earth

- ability to keep your own ego in check

- commitment to remaining healthy yourself, through wise lifestyle choices and ideally also through the pursuit of energy arts such as Qi Gong or Tai Chi.

If you diligently practise all of the above, there should be little risk of damaging either yourself or your clients in any way. Washing your hands under cold running water is also very beneficial after each and every treatment. I also recommend going for a walk in the fresh air between clients, if this is practical. These things really do help.

Vulnerable patients

It is also very important to bear in mind that certain individuals fall into the 'vulnerable' category as far as healing goes. Those with a terminal illness or mental ill health or those who are extremely debilitated require extra consideration, for your sake as much as theirs. The Qi of such individuals is often fragile or chaotic. In these cases, fine judgement needs to be applied as to how much healing to give, or, occasionally, even whether to give it at all. Sometimes it is best to fall back on your existing therapy. This does not reflect any judgement on the patient, but rather a concern for their wellbeing. As usual, if in doubt – don't.

Now let's look at some case studies to gain further insight into how you might integrate QSH into your existing therapy routines in the clinic. Please note that the diagnostic portion of each of these studies has been deliberately simplified. This is to avoid becoming bogged down in the terminology of any particular style. Therefore the diagnosis laid out at the beginning of each study is not couched specifically in terms of TCM, five-element Acupuncture, Tui Na or any other modality. Instead, it will simply give an outline of the patient's tendency to imbalance in the general terms of Chinese Medicine. Studies will also contain basic Western anatomical and medical references. References to 'pulse taking' refer, of course, to the Chinese, not Western, concept of how energetic imbalances can be detected via the pulse.

Case Study A: Qi Sensitivity Healing plus Traditional Chinese Medicine Acupuncture

Female, mid-30s.

Main complaint (Western)

Sinusitis, principally in the frontal sinuses, of two weeks' duration. This complaint appears to have followed on from a lingering viral infection that has also left the patient with a hacking cough and considerable mucus. The patient has been undergoing significant and ongoing personal stress and describes herself as generally run-down and exhausted. Muscle tension in the neck, shoulders and upper back. No previous history of sinusitis. No medications, other than self-prescribed decongestants and mild painkillers.

Simplified diagnosis (Traditional Chinese, from pulse and tongue analysis)

Principal imbalance: an excess in Stomach Meridian, alongside deficient Spleen Meridian. Underlying Kidney, Heart and Pericardium Meridian Qi deficiencies. Overall Qi deficiency and stagnation. Phlegm. Shen slightly disturbed.

QSH diagnosis

Considerable activity around the entire head, with particularly 'sticky', stagnant Qi perceived in EEF above forehead. Weak or 'empty' areas in EEF manifesting around lower Dan Tien and localized on right leg at acupoint Zu San Li (ST 36). A generally 'chaotic' Qi sensation around the area of the heart.

Treatment

Acupuncture: Needles retained at acupoints on Stomach and Spleen Meridians, plus various local points in forehead.

QSH

With needles in situ, De Qi with the earth is obtained with the left hand, with the right hand held approximately four inches above the patient's forehead. 'Pulling threads' and a 'Smoothing out' technique are applied around the head for approximately five minutes. The patient reports a sudden alleviation of pain in her sinuses.

'Hovering palm' technique is now employed over the middle, then lower Dan Tien. Then the 'Sensing finger' technique is used on the right-sided acupoint Zu San Li. Finally, the patient's feet are lightly grasped in 'Distal grip' technique to provide grounding, for two minutes. She reports feelings of 'lightness' and 'unusual calm'. Her sinus pain is much reduced.

The needles are now removed and the patient's pulse re-checked. There is a distinct improvement in the strength and quality of the pulse throughout, particularly on the Stomach and Spleen Meridians. Palpation also shows a significant reduction in muscular tension, even in areas that have not been directly treated.

Note: If this was solely an Acupuncture treatment, I would tend to end the session with more needling to tonify (strengthen) the weakest meridians. In this case it is deemed unnecessary, as pulse diagnosis and verbal feedback from the patient suggests strongly that QSH has already achieved this aim throughout her entire energy system.

Case Study B: Qi Sensitivity
Healing plus Tui Na Massage
Female, mid-70s.

Main complaint (Western)

This lady is generally robust and healthy, but likes to have regular Tui Na massage as part of a general preventative health care programme. She is also a carer for a disabled relative and finds massage a great stress-reliever. Today there is considerable muscle tension and mild pain from trigger points around the right scapula, and especially between the scapula and spine. Palpation also reveals some discomfort around the posterior head of the deltoid. She reports feeling rather tired.

Simplified diagnosis (Traditional Chinese,
from pulse and tongue analysis)

Localized stagnation of Blood and Qi, especially in areas of Small Intestine and Bladder Meridians referring to scapula and upper back. The Small Intestine Meridian is possibly implicated in the deltoid issue. There is some degree of generalized Qi and Yin deficiency throughout the system, principally manifesting in Kidney Meridian.

QSH diagnosis

Generally coherent Qi throughout the EEF, although some 'dark' or 'stagnant' energy is located in specific, highly localized locations on the patient's back and shoulders.

The right side is worst, but similar points are also located on the left side of the upper body.

These locations are principally acupoints on the Bladder and Small Intestine Meridians, but several are in the Ahshi (trigger point) category and not meridian-related. Rather than an overall deficiency of Qi, a general impression is arrived at of a very slight but perceptible 'sluggishness' within the entire energy system.

QSH treatment

QSH is applied prior to any massage in this example. This choice has been made to mobilize the patient's Qi and to 'soften her up' in terms of relaxation. This is done in the expectation that the duration of the massage can be significantly shortened. Moreover, invasive deep-tissue work on painful areas can be kept to an absolute minimum or even dispensed with altogether.

With the patient on her back on the treatment couch, the therapist's hands are slipped under her upper back bilaterally either side of the spine where the pain is perceived, for five minutes.

Many acupoints are covered in this way, and once a feeling of healthy energetic 'opening' and 'vibration' is achieved throughout the area, the therapist's hands are moved to cover the general scapula area for five minutes, and then the entire deltoid areas, for approximately three minutes.

Right-sided acupoint Jian Zhen (SI 9) seems to require extra work, and so the 'Sensing finger' technique is applied for two minutes.

Tui Na whole-body massage is now employed for approximately 20 minutes using a broad range of standard Traditional Chinese Massage techniques. Any particular emphasis on Massage/Acupressure of acupoints and formerly painful areas around the right scapula, deltoid and upper back is now redundant. The patient enjoys a thorough but pain-free massage and reports feeling more mobile and invigorated by the end of the session. A re-taking of the pulse plus a QSH body scan reveals a welcome increase in the overall vitality of the meridian system.

Case Study C: Qi Sensitivity Healing
plus five-element style Acupuncture

Male, early 50s.

Main complaint (Western)
Metastatic liver cancer, currently held in check by an ongoing chemotherapy regime.

Previous history of prostate cancer. Chemo is proving effective in shrinking and containing multiple tumours so far, but is having a devastating effect on the patient's general health. Hair loss, deep fatigue, insomnia, constant nausea and sporadic depression are all present. Other medications are now being taken to attempt to combat some of these issues.

Simplified diagnosis (Traditional Chinese)
This patient is a vocal advocate of J.R. Worsley-style, five-element Acupuncture.[1] After discussion, a close examination of the patient's pulse, tongue, signs and symptoms leads us to the conclusion that absolutely any intervention must be minimal, due to the overall levels of debilitation. We decide together that a judicious mixture of five-element Acupuncture and QSH is appropriate. In the language of the five-element modality, I diagnose the patient's fundamental imbalance as belonging to the Wood element. There is also a noticeable knock-on effect of this basic imbalance in the Earth and Fire element levels of his being. The Heart and Pericardium Meridians feel particularly 'empty' to a QSH scan. The patient, normally a vivacious and colourful character, expresses his chief wish as 'losing this miserable depression'. He feels the medical profession is dealing well with his physical symptoms, but wishes me to intervene on a more subtle, energetic/emotional level.

Minimal Acupuncture is applied to points along the Liver and Gall Bladder Meridians to re-establish flow between these meridians and those of the Earth element. This seems to have an almost immediate effect both on the patient's nausea and on the strength and quality of Qi in the system as a whole.

QSH

I now select acupoint Ji Quan (HT 1) for 'Sensing finger' with my right hand, whilst wrapping my entire left hand around the same-side little finger as a distal location. I wait until I feel the meridian 'open', then I switch to the other side of his body. He reports feeling unaccountably 'more cheerful', even 'exultant' (his words). However, he now complains of a sudden feeling of heaviness and discomfort around the general area of the solar plexus. I employ 'Knife hand' technique to allow this to dissipate safely down the front of his body, whilst establishing De Qi with the ground with 'Dropped finger' technique.

We both deem this to be enough treatment for today. It would be all too easy to exhaust him.

The patient is now feeling calm but happy, and reports a general cessation of nausea and fatigue, at least for now.

In terms of energy hygiene, this particular case demands that I check and re-check the patient's energy system by constantly stopping to scan with one hand over his EEF. I am looking for any sign that his energy is being depleted or made less coherent by my treatment.

At the same time, I am very keen to ground both of us by at all times maintaining De Qi with the earth with either 'Dropped finger' technique and/or via the soles of my feet. I also make sure that he is not draining me, and pay special attention to sensations of Qi being pulled out and away from me. In this case there are none; otherwise I might eschew QSH and just provide him with a very simple, minimalist Acupuncture treatment. Safety first, for both parties!

Case Study D: Qi Sensitivity Healing
as a stand-alone therapy

Female, early 40s.

Main complaint (Western)

No specific illness as such, just a general feeling of being constantly 'under the weather'.

There is also ongoing stress in her personal life that causes mild anxiety symptoms such as palpitations and insomnia. The patient has tight musculature, especially around the shoulders and upper back, and sometimes suffers from IBS-type symptoms. Her menses have also become slightly irregular.

Simplified diagnosis, QSH-style

A QSH scan of the EEF shows significant depletion of this woman's energy. There are palpable 'holes' in her EEF, especially above the lower Dan Tien, which also feels cold to the touch, even through clothing. There is also a feeling of a certain lumpen 'heaviness' to her Qi in general. The exception to this is around her head, which feels 'electric' but not in any way balanced. I notice that both her feet are very cold too.

QSH treatment

Using an entire range of QSH techniques, as intuition dictates, I attempt to (a) repair the holes in the EEF, (b) make the Qi in and around her head descend safely down the front of the body to the lower Dan Tien, and (c) ground her energy by holding her feet. I also open specific acupoints/meridians whenever I find them blocked or dysfunctional, especially on and around the spine. Please note, however, that this is not a treatment plan as such. In fact, nothing is planned whatsoever. What unfolds during our hour-long session simply happens according to what I perceive to be the state of her Qi at any given moment, and also according to verbal feedback from the patient herself. I spend half an hour treating the back of her body, and then I ask her to turn over on the treatment couch to enable the front of the body to be accessed.

By the end of the treatment this patient is feeling much calmer and more relaxed. She also notices a substantial improvement in her physical flexibility and overall bodily warmth. She says she feels 'balanced' for the first time in weeks.

Some final thoughts…

Obviously, the four case studies that I have given here are far from definitive. They merely scratch the surface of the potential of QSH, either used in conjunction with other therapies or as a stand-alone treatment. Be creative; experiment! However, never lose sight of the fact that you have a care of duty to your patients, and that any experimenting you undertake must always be carried out with their interests uppermost in your mind at all times. This book has given you the tools to do that. Good luck!

Notes

1.   The late J.R. Worsley was a noted British acupuncturist whose name has become synonymous with the introduction of five-element style Chinese Medicine to the West.

References

Kornfield, J. (2002) *A Path with Heart*. London: Rider Books, p.62.

Mitchell, D. (2013) *Heavenly Streams: Meridian Theory in Nei Gong*. London: Singing Dragon, p.21.

Villoldo, A. (2001) *Shaman, Healer, Sage: How to Heal Yourself and Others with the Energy Medicine of the Americas*. London: Bantam Books, p.43.

Watts, A. (1992) *Tao: The Watercourse Way*. London: Penguin Arkana, p.76.

Further Reading

Daoism (general)

Cleary, T. (trans., ed.) (1991) *Vitality, Energy, Spirit: A Taoist Sourcebook.* Boston, MA and London: Shambhala Dragon Editions.

Freke, T. (ed.) (1995) *Lao Tzu's Tao Te Ching.* London: Piatkus Publishing.

Hinton, D. (2012) *Hunger Mountain.* Boston, MA and London: Shambhala Dragon Editions.

Huan, Z.Y. and Rose, K. (1999) *Who Can Ride the Dragon? An Exploration of the Cultural Roots of Traditional Chinese Medicine.* Brookline, MA: Paradigm Publications.

I-Ming, L. (1988) *Awakening to the Tao* (Translated by Thomas Clearly). Boston, MA and London: Shambhala Dragon Editions.

Kaiguo, C. and Shunchao, Z. (1996) *Opening the Dragon Gate: The Making of a Modern Daoist Wizard* (Translated by Thomas Clearly). Boston, MA: Tuttle Publishing.

Ming-Dao, D. (1990) *Scholar Warrior: An Introduction to the Dao in Everyday Life.* New York: HarperCollins.

Watts, A. (1999) *Taoism: Way Beyond Seeking, The Edited Manuscripts.* London: Thorsons (HarperCollins).

Wong, E. (1995) *Lieh-Tzu: A Taoist Guide to Practical Living.* Boston, MA: Shambhala Dragon Editions.

Qi Gong and Nei Gong

Cohen, K.S. (1997) *The Way of Qigong: The Art and Science of Chinese Energy Healing.* London: Bantam Books.

Frantzis, B.K. (1993) *Opening the Energy Gates of Your Body: Gain Lifelong Vitality.* Berkeley, CA: North Atlantic Books.

Mitchell, D. (2011) *Daoist Nei Gong: The Philosophical Art of Change.* London and Philadelphia, PA: Singing Dragon.

Ni, H.-C. (1997) *Entering the Tao: Master Ni's Guidance for Self-Cultivation.* Boston, MA: Shambhala Publications.

Reid, S. (1997) *Guarding the Three Treasures: The Chinese Way of Health.* London: Simon & Schuster UK.

Wu, Z. (2008) *Vital Breath of the Dao: Chinese Shamanic Tiger Qigong – Laohu Gong.* London: Singing Dragon.

External Qi Healing (EQH)

Johnson, J.A. (2000) *Chinese Medical Qigong Therapy: A Comprehensive Clinical Text* (Edited by Jampa Mackenzie Stewart and Madeleine H. Howell). Pacific Grove, CA: The International Institute of Medical Qigong.

Yongsheng, B. (1992) *Chinese Qigong Outgoing-Qi Therapy* (Translated by Yu Wenping). Jinan, China: Shandong Science and Technology Press.

Meridians and Acupoint location

Jiasan, Y. (ed.) (1982) *The Way to Locate Acupoints* (Translated by Dr Meng Xiankun and Dr Li Xuewu). Beijing: Foreign Language Press.

Ogal, H.P. and Stor, W. (eds) (2005) *Pictorial Atlas of Acupuncture: An Illustrated Manual of Acupuncture Points.* Marburg, Germany: Ullmann Publishing.

Acupuncture and Traditional Chinese Medicine (TCM)

Benfield, H. and Korngold, E. (1991) *Between Heaven and Earth: A Guide to Chinese Medicine.* New York: Ballantine Wellspring, (Ballantine Publishing).

Connelly, D.M. (1979) *Traditional Acupuncture: The Law of the Five Elements.* Towson, MD: The Center for Traditional Acupuncture.

Maciocia, G. (1989) *The Foundations of Chinese Medicine: A Comprehensive Text for Acupuncturists and Herbalists.* Edinburgh, London, Melbourne and New York: Churchill Livingstone.

Reichstein, G. (1998) *Wood Becomes Water: Chinese Medicine in Everyday Life.* New York, Tokyo and London: Kodansha International.

Hands-on healing, general

Brennan, B.A. (1987) *Hands of Light: A Guide to Healing Through the Human Energy Field.* New York: Bantam Books.

Brennan, B.A. (1993) *Light Emerging: A Journey of Personal Healing.* New York: Bantam Books.

Burmeister, A. with Monte, T. (1997) *Practical Jin Shin Jyutsu: Energise Your Body, Mind and Spirit the Traditional Japanese Way.* New York: Bantam Books.

Tui Na (Chinese Massage)

Jianguo, F., Xueqin, G., Liangyi, Z., Xiaoning, L. and Shuchun, S. (chief ed.) (1989) *Atlas of Therapeutic Motion for Treatment and Health – A Guide to Traditional Chinese Massage and Exercise Therapy* (Translated by Chen Baoxing, Li Jinxue and Wei Yuanping). Beijing: Foreign Languages Press.

Pritchard, S. (1999) *Chinese Massage Manual: A Comprehensive Step-By-Step Guide to the Healing Art of Tui Na*. London: Piatkus Publishers Ltd.

Appendix

Acupoints

HT 1 In the centre of the axilla (armpit), just medial to the axillary artery.

PC 6 2 cun above the wrist crease, between the tendons of palmaris longus and flexor carpi radialis.

PC 8 On the palm between the bones of the 2nd and 3rd metacarpals. Roughly where the curled ring finger touches the palm.

SI 9 On the back of the shoulder, 1 cun above the axillary fold.

GB 20 On the back of the neck, 1 cun above the hairline, halfway between the midline of the neck and the lower edge of the mastoid process.

KD1 On the midline of the sole of the foot, in a hollow approximately one-third of the distance between the base of the toes and the heel.

KD 7 Approximately 0.4 cun in a direct line below the lower border of the medial malleolus (ankle bone).

LV 3 On the front of the foot, between the first and second metatarsals, just distal to where the two bones meet.

ST 36 On the upper shin, one finger-width lateral to the edge of the tibia, at the distal edge of the tibial tuberosity (bulge).

ST40 On the shin, 8 cun above the tip of the lateral malleolus (ankle bone), 2 finger-widths lateral to the crest of the tibia.

ST 41 On the midline of the ankle crease, between the large tendons of extensor digitorum longus, and extensor hallucis longus.

SP 4　On the medial side of the foot, just distal and inferior to the bulge of the 1st metatarsal.

UB10　On the back of the neck, approximately 1.5 cun lateral to the midline, just above the hairline.

UB12　On the upper back, 1.5 cun lateral to the midline of the spine, inferior to the tip of the spinous process of T2.

CV 1　In a hollow on the midline of the perineum, half way between the anus and the lower edge of the genitals.

CV15　On the midline of the body, below the ribcage, 1 cun inferior to the xiphoid process.

GV4　On the midline of the spine, just below the tip of the process of the L2 vertebra.

Ren Mai　The meridian that flows down the midline of the front of the body.

GV20　On the crown of the head, on the midline, on a line connecting the tips of both ears.

Du Mai　The meridian that flows up the midline of the back of the body.

Chong Mai　The meridian that runs through the core of the body, connecting the crown of the head with the perineum.

HN 5　Taiyang: In a hollow on the side of the head, 1 cun posterior to the lateral edge of the eyebrow ridge and the outer canthus of the eye.

B2 Hua Tuo Jia Ji　A series of 17 acupoints on the back, between L5 and T1; 1.5 cun lateral to the midline of the spine, in the hollow formed by the spinous process of each vertebra.

Index

Rob Long is an experienced Acupuncturist, Tui Na therapist and Qi Gong healer and teacher. Based in Cornwall, Rob has been offering clients and students clinical work and teaching based on in-depth knowledge of traditional Daoist skills for two decades.

CPI Antony Rowe
Eastbourne, UK
January 05, 2024